Hysterectomy

Janet Wright is the author of 11 books on healthy living. Her work has been translated into more than a dozen languages, sold around the world WRI and commended by the Medical Journalists' Association. A graduate of University College London, she specializes in finding treatments and self-help techniques backed by reliable evidence. Her previous book for Sheldon was *Coping with Perimenopause* (2006).

Overcoming Common Problems Series

Selected titles

A full list of titles is available from Sheldon Press,
36 Causton Street, London SW1P 4ST and on our website at
www.sheldonpress.co.uk

Backache: What you need to know
Dr David Delvin

The Cancer Survivor's Handbook
Dr Terry Priestman

The Chronic Pain Diet Book
Neville Shone

Coping Successfully with Psoriasis
Christine Craggs-Hinton

Coping When Your Child Has Cerebral Palsy
Jill Eckersley

Coping with Birth Trauma and Postnatal Depression
Lucy Jolin

Coping with Chemotherapy
Dr Terry Priestman

Coping with Epilepsy in Children and Young People
Susan Elliot-Wright

Coping with Hay Fever
Christine Craggs-Hinton

Coping with Headaches and Migraine
Alison Frith

Coping with Kidney Disease
Dr Tom Smith

Coping with Life after Stroke
Dr Mareeni Raymond

Coping with PMS
Dr Farah Ahmed and Dr Emma Cordle

Coping with Polycystic Ovary Syndrome
Christine Craggs-Hinton

Coping with Type 2 Diabetes
Susan Elliot-Wright

Coping with Your Partner's Death: Your bereavement guide
Geoff Billings

Every Woman's Guide to Digestive Health
Jill Eckersley

The Fibromyalgia Healing Diet
Christine Craggs-Hinton

Free Yourself from Depression
Colin and Margaret Sutherland

A Guide to Anger Management
Mary Hartley

How to Fight Chronic Fatigue
Christine Craggs-Hinton

Hysterectomy: Is it right for you?
Janet Wright

Living with Angina
Dr Tom Smith

Living with Bipolar Disorder
Dr Neel Burton

Living with Gluten Intolerance
Jane Feinmann

Living with Physical Disability and Amputation
Dr Keren Fisher

Living with Type 1 Diabetes
Dr Tom Smith

Osteoporosis: Prevent and treat
Dr Tom Smith

Overcome Your Fear of Flying
Professor Robert Bor, Dr Carina Eriksen and Margaret Oakes

Overcoming Agoraphobia
Melissa Murphy

Overcoming Insomnia
Susan Elliot-Wright

Overcoming Panic and Related Anxiety Disorders
Margaret Hawkins

Overcoming Shyness and Social Anxiety
Ruth Searle

Overcoming Tiredness and Exhaustion
Fiona Marshall

Reducing Your Risk of Cancer
Dr Terry Priestman

Safe Dieting for Teens
Linda Ojeda

Self-discipline: How to get it and how to keep it
Dr Windy Dryden

Sinusitis: Steps to healing
Dr Paul Carson

Stammering: Advice for all ages
Renée Byrne and Louise Wright

When Someone You Love Has Dementia
Susan Elliot-Wright

Overcoming Common Problems

Hysterectomy: Is It Right for You?

JANET WRIGHT

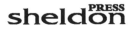

First published in Great Britain in 2009

Sheldon Press
36 Causton Street
London SW1P 4ST

British Library Cataloguing-in-Publication Data
A catalogue record for this book is available from the British Library

ISBN 978-1-84709-051-5

1 3 5 7 9 10 8 6 4 2

Typeset by Fakenham Photosetting Ltd, Fakenham, Norfolk
Printed in Great Britain by Ashford Colour Press

Produced on paper from sustainable forests

Contents

To all the women who have helped with my research over the years, and to David Hall for everything.

1

Introduction

Hysterectomy is an operation to remove the uterus, or womb. It will cure problems caused by the uterus itself and has a good chance of curing those caused by the menstrual cycle. It's necessary to save your life if you have certain forms of cancer. But it means you can no longer have children. Your menopause is likely to come sooner than if you had not had the operation, and you may have other side effects.

If you're thinking about hysterectomy and its alternatives, you're probably experiencing symptoms of a gynaecological condition. Perhaps you've had a diagnosis, and your doctor has suggested the possibility of removing your uterus. Or perhaps you're generously doing the research for a friend or relative, as the shock of a diagnosis can leave people feeling bewildered about the right path to take.

You're wise to look into the options, because there are many more available now than even a few years ago. There is also a wealth of self-help advice. See later chapters of this book for the many ways you can ease your symptoms, reduce your risk of a recurrence, and even possibly avoid the need for an operation.

Hysterectomy is a very common procedure. Every year some 40,000 women have one in the United Kingdom. In the United States the number is at least 600,000 – about a third of all US women have lost their uterus before the age of 60. Only a few decades ago, a hysterectomy was the first choice of treatment for all kinds of conditions. Some gynaecologists even considered that the uterus was unnecessary after a woman had passed child-bearing age, and should be removed in case it caused trouble!

Thankfully, those days are past. In fact, if you're under 40 it may be hard to imagine an era when a doctor could openly express such views. In tune with the changing times, the number of hysterectomies carried out each year is falling, especially in the UK and mainland Europe, as alternatives become more widely known. Women are likely to be offered less invasive alternatives for most conditions.

That doesn't mean a hysterectomy is never the answer. It would be foolish to rule out an operation that can cure painful or disabling conditions, if all else fails. But it is major surgery, and some of its effects may be unwelcome, especially if you are still young. You may still wish to have children, and an early menopause can bring problems of its own. There are many other routes worth considering, if the condition is not life-threatening and you have time to consider alternatives.

Diagnosis

First, it is important to get a diagnosis for your symptoms. Gynaecological conditions can cause a host of vague symptoms – including intermittent pain, bleeding, discomfort, and bladder irritation. It's hard to know, at first, whether they're important or not. But that is the time when you need to have them checked out.

If the cause is something serious, such as cancer, you have a good chance of successful treatment if it's been diagnosed in the early stages. If it's something minor but annoying, you have time to browse through treatment options.

Non-cancerous conditions that may lead to a hysterectomy include:

- heavy periods (menorrhagia)
- very painful periods (dysmenorrhoea)
- growths such as fibroids, adenomyomas and polyps
- endometriosis: cells from inside the womb growing out of place, around the other organs
- pelvic inflammatory disease (PID)
- endometrial hyperplasia: pre-cancerous changes to the womb lining
- premenstrual syndrome (PMS)
- prolapsed womb: when the uterus sags into the vagina.

Self-help

Lifestyle changes can help a great deal, before you even begin to look at therapies. Even if you go on to follow the orthodox route, these do-it-yourself techniques should provide valuable back-up. And they can often reduce your risk of the problem flaring up again.

Many kinds of physical activity ease the pain caused by long-term conditions. But it can be hard to take exercise when you're held back by pain or torrential bleeding. The answer is to tailor an exercise routine to meet your individual needs and your current capabilities. Particular exercises have been devised to tackle specific problems: Kegel exercises, for example, can tone up the pelvic-floor muscles that hold the uterus in place, easing the dragging discomfort caused when it starts to sag.

Likewise, nutritional help goes beyond just healthy eating, useful though that is. Certain foods can reduce the hormonal upheaval that lies behind many gynaecological problems. Or they can relieve symptoms: eating iron-rich ingredients can counteract the iron loss caused by heavy bleeding, for example. Others can make your symptoms worse. This book shows you how to find out what's likely to be causing a problem and how to avoid it.

Professional help

There's a bewildering variety of options. The internet can come up with a hundred remedies for any condition you care to name. And when the condition is serious enough to warrant major surgery, people may feel motivated to try anything that promises an easier cure. But how do you work out what's genuine, and what's likely to help you? Read on to find out.

Complementary therapies have much to offer some women whose conditions don't necessitate orthodox treatment, or as a back-up to relieve symptoms. Something as simple as massage can ease the backache caused by painful periods. Many people have tried acupuncture or acupressure. And herbal remedies are widely used. See later chapters for advice and evidence about their effectiveness.

The medical profession also has many more options these days. No longer do women face the harsh choice of a full hysterectomy or nothing. Many medicines and other treatments have been developed to solve gynaecological problems that once kept women in a state of ill-health for decades.

Hormonal drugs (including the contraceptive Pill) have eased many women's gynaecological problems, especially those connected with periods. Other drugs can be used if the hormones don't help. Even antibiotics have a role to play, when used correctly.

As a next step, there are several minor operations that can remove growths, for example, without harming the uterus itself. Fibroids and other non-cancerous growths can be cut out. Where the womb lining has grown out of place, it can be cut out or burnt off with a laser.

Surgeons can operate using tiny cameras and equipment on flexible tubes that enter your abdomen through the smallest of incisions. In some cases, they can work up through the vagina, so you don't have any scar at all.

With non-urgent conditions (and that's most of them) there's no reason not to start with self-help, or the least invasive procedure. You can always progress to the next stage if the first is not successful, or if it is only enough to hold the problem at bay for a while.

Options in hysterectomy

Some conditions, however, will not respond to minor operations or self-help. Painful periods or heavy bleeding, for example, sometimes persist despite all efforts to alleviate them, as long as your womb is still in place. And if you've been diagnosed with cancer of the uterus, you almost certainly will be advised to have a hysterectomy without delay.

If you do need to have a hysterectomy, this can take several forms. It can often be done using the same minimally invasive methods mentioned above: entering through the vagina or via a tiny incision. The smallest procedure leaves the cervix intact; the biggest removes the ovaries and some other tissue as well as the whole uterus.

After a hysterectomy, there is much you can do for yourself to aid recovery, and improve the chance of a long-term solution to your health problems. If your ovaries have been removed, causing a sudden menopause, you may consider using hormone replacement therapy (HRT). But many women have been put off HRT by news that it increases the risk of several diseases, notably breast cancer. It's worth checking the evidence as it relates to your particular circumstances, and considering the alternatives.

This book looks at all the options, from self-help to cutting-edge treatments. It provides some ideas on what is most likely to be helpful in different conditions, and how to use it safely and effectively.

Throughout this book, 'hysterectomy' means the removal of the womb. It doesn't include removal of the ovaries unless that is stated. Included at the back of the book is a Glossary explaining medical conditions and procedures referred to through the book.

Don't give cancer a chance to grow

Cancer is an exception to the rule of starting with the mildest treatment first. Please don't waste any time if you have been diagnosed with cancer and advised to have a hysterectomy. By all means get a second opinion if you wish, from a medical specialist who can advise on how much needs to be removed, and whether you'll need chemotherapy or radiotherapy. But don't delay in the hope of finding an alternative remedy. Cancer can spread rapidly and should be taken out as quickly as possible.

There is no evidence that any non-mainstream therapy can cure any kind of cancer.

2

The inside story

Like so much else about the human body, the reproductive system is a seemingly simple mechanism that's kept running by an amazingly complex support network. The simple-looking part is the anatomy of your uterus and the surrounding organs. The complex part is how it all works, largely through the action of hormones.

Because gynaecological (women's) problems often affect other parts of the abdomen, it's useful to know roughly where everything is.

Your body

From the outside, you can see your external sex organs more clearly by holding a mirror to your groin. Your pubic hair grows on the outer lips, or labia majora. The area that can be seen when you part your pubic hair is the vulva.

Looking downwards from the top the first thing you can see, or feel, is the little bump of the clitoris. Next comes the opening to the urethra, through which urine leaves the body. Next is the vaginal opening. On each side of this are the inner lips, or labia minora, looking like a frill of loose flesh. These are often uneven in size and shape, and vary greatly in appearance from one woman to the next. Then the perineum, a smooth expanse of skin, continues until it reaches the anus, through which solid waste leaves your body.

Inside your abdomen, your uterus is about the size and shape of an upside-down pear. It expands enormously, of course, during pregnancy, but usually returns to its previous size after childbirth. This ability to spring back into shape is aided by a thick layer of muscle called the myometrium; inside that is the inner layer, or endometrium. (The outer layer is called the perimetrium.) At the top, the two fallopian tubes lead to the uterus from the left and right ovaries. At the bottom, the uterus narrows into the cervix, which is the mouth of the womb.

Continuing downwards from the cervix, like a long hollow 'stalk' from the pear, is the vagina, which leads to the outside of the body. During sexual intercourse the man's penis enters the vagina, and during childbirth the baby is pushed headfirst down it into the world.

Close to the uterus are the liver, kidneys, stomach and other internal organs. Metres of intestine are coiled inside the abdomen, digesting your food along the way from the stomach to the bowel. Urine passes from your kidneys along tubes called ureters into the bladder, where it is held – under your control – until you are ready to urinate; then it leaves your body through another tube called the urethra.

There are many connections among all these organs. The uterus, for example, is held in place by strap-like ligaments joining it to the bladder and the rectum, the last part of the intestine. Looking at how it all fits in together, it's not surprising that when something happens to the uterus it can affect other processes such as your digestion or your ability to control urination.

Your hormones

The gynaecological conditions that lead women to consider having a hysterectomy are often caused by something going wrong with the reproductive hormones.

Hormones are chemicals that carry instructions from one part of the body to another, travelling in the bloodstream. Produced by glands in various different organs, including the brain and the ovaries, they play a major role in many of the body's systems, all aimed at keeping it functioning smoothly.

Some are meant for emergencies: adrenaline, for example, speeds up the heart and tells the liver to release energy-giving glucose into your bloodstream, fuelling you to either run or fight for your life. Sometimes hormones slip out of balance, causing conditions such as diabetes (not enough insulin) or an underactive or overactive thyroid (the wrong amount of thyroid hormones).

No one except a medical expert needs to know the names of the many hormones that keep our hearts beating, our digestive systems working, our fluid levels constant and so on. The hormones most of us could name are involved in the reproductive system: *oestrogen, progesterone, testosterone*. Those are the main players in this book.

Note: Watch out for alternative spellings if you're using the internet for research. US spelling doesn't use the 'oe' at the beginning of words such as oestrogen, which is spelt 'estrogen'. Gonadotrophin is 'gonadotropin' in US usage. Progestogen is sometimes spelt progestagen.

Some non-reproductive hormones may also play a role in gynaecological conditions, because of the complex interplay between them and the hormones that govern our reproductive system, especially oestrogen.

Insulin in high levels has been linked with uterine (womb) cancer, so there's a chance that it may also play a role in other oestrogen-fuelled conditions such as fibroids and endometriosis.

High levels of oestrogen may reduce the effectiveness of certain *thyroid* hormones. An underactive thyroid is a condition that needs treating in itself, but it may also be a clue that oestrogen levels are excessively high.

Stress hormones – which our bodies produce more of when we're anxious or pressured – such as *cortisol* have a powerfully disruptive effect on the reproductive hormones. They have been linked with many gynaecological conditions including fibroids.

The reproductive system

Like almost everything in the complex organism of our bodies, reproductive hormones play many roles, large and small. They may even affect our minds, by influencing production of chemicals called neurotransmitters that affect our emotions and brainpower. But their major role is to regulate our menstrual cycles and pregnancies. Throughout this book, most references to 'hormones' mean reproductive hormones.

The two best-known reproductive hormones are oestrogen and progesterone, which play different roles in pregnancy and the menstrual cycle, largely by balancing each other's actions. Their levels fluctuate throughout our lives, most noticeably at puberty, throughout pregnancy and for some time after birth, and during the menopause. But we are also producing different levels of hormones during every menstrual cycle (see below).

Many factors, from anxiety to dieting, can affect hormone production enough to throw it off balance. And some women are just more sensitive than others to hormonal changes. Many women have experienced mood swings, tiredness or food cravings just before a period is due. Some women have it badly enough to be diagnosed with premenstrual syndrome (PMS).

Oestrogen (or 'estrogen' in the US spelling) plays the biggest role in our reproductive life. It occurs in three slightly different forms. The two minor ones are oestrone (or estrone, or E1), which is still produced in small amounts by fat cells after the menopause, and oestriol (estriol, E3), the weakest form, only produced in the placenta during pregnancy. Oestradiol (estradiol, E2) is the main form, produced by the ovaries throughout our reproductive life. It helps prepare for pregnancy.

Progestogens are a group of hormones including progesterone, the one we produce most throughout our lives. The word 'progestogen' is also used for the synthetic forms used in contraceptives and other hormonal drugs; these are also sometimes called 'progestins'. In common usage (and in this book unless otherwise stated) 'progesterone' means the form that we produce naturally and 'progestogen' means the synthetic version.

Progesterone is released after ovulation and starts preparing the womb lining for a pregnancy. If a fertilized egg is implanted, a different form of progestogen works throughout the pregnancy to keep it safe. But if not, the womb lining is sloughed off, a period starts and the menstrual cycle begins again. Progesterone can be converted into other hormones when they're needed, including oestrogen.

Testosterone (among other androgens, or 'male hormones') plays many roles in women's bodies. In the right amounts, testosterone provides energy and sex drive, but in excess it can cause aggression. Production peaks twice in the menstrual cycle: first around the time of ovulation, increasing our sex drive at the best time for conception, and again just before a period is due, when it can fuel PMS. Levels fall as you reach the menopause.

Follicle-stimulating hormone (FSH) helps the ovaries bring an egg to maturity each month. It is only produced in large quantities when there isn't much oestrogen in the body. A high FSH level is normal during the first week of the menstrual cycle, and after the menopause. At other times, in women who are still having periods, it could mean a lack of oestrogen – a possible warning of premature menopause. Low FSH levels can cause your periods to stop.

Luteinizing hormone (LH) causes the ovary to release the egg when it is ready to be fertilized. During our fertile years, LH levels are usually low except around the time of ovulation. As with FSH, high LH levels can be a warning of early menopause.

Human chorionic gonadotrophin (HCG) starts being produced in the placenta soon after an egg is fertilized. It stimulates the ovaries to produce more oestrogen and progesterone to support the pregnancy.

Gonadotrophin releasing hormone (GnRH), also known as luteinizing hormone releasing hormone (LHRH), stimulates the pituitary gland to produce FSH and LH, especially just before ovulation. Drugs opposing the effects of GnRH may be used to treat gynaecological conditions.

The two faces of oestrogen

More than any other hormone, oestrogen is what makes us recognizably female, and what gives us the ability to have and nurture babies. It plays many other roles, keeping our hearts and bones strong and even helping us to get to sleep at night.

But essential though it is, oestrogen has an important downside. In excess, or when it's out of balance with other hormones, oestrogen causes many of the conditions that may lead to a hysterectomy. It's what causes heavy bleeding and painful periods. It promotes the growth of things you don't want, such as fibroids, endometriosis, polyps and cancers including those of the uterus, cervix and ovaries. Many of the treatments in this book, both orthodox and self-help, are aimed at countering the harmful effects of oestrogen.

Why does this vital hormone turn against us? There are many theories. One is that we just live longer than our ancestors did, giving all the body's systems more time to go wrong – and the most powerful systems cause the most harm.

Do women suffer from more hormonal conditions these days, or do we just know more about them? Up until recent centuries, people wouldn't have known what was going wrong inside – they would just become ill or die. And with so many infectious diseases and so few medicines, not to mention the high risk of dying in childbirth, few women would have survived long enough to die of cancer.

However, we are heavier, on average, than even our grandmothers' generation, and considerably more than our distant ancestors throughout the millions of years of evolution. Fat cells produce a small amount of oestrogen, even after the menopause. So throughout life, the heavier we are, the higher our oestrogen levels are likely to be. Well into the twentieth century, people were more likely to starve to death than to suffer health conditions related to body fat.

Also, we now breathe in or consume a cocktail of chemicals that didn't exist a hundred years ago. Many of these man-made chemicals, found in everyday items or as by-products of industry, are now known to have oestrogenic effects. Known as 'xenoestrogens', they have been linked with reproductive cancers in women and low sperm counts in men. See later chapters on lifestyle and nutrition for information on how to avoid them.

Yet gynaecological conditions strike women of all sizes and ages. Being slim is no guarantee of freedom from menstrual disorders, and being underweight promotes different hormonal problems. Some women are just more sensitive than others to hormonal changes, including the effects of oestrogen. That's the reason why, even if all hormone tests seem normal, we may have hormone-related problems. It's just part of our individual physical make-up.

Life cycles

Puberty

Girls are born with hundreds of thousands of minuscule eggs in tiny sacs called follicles, inside the ovaries. These stay dormant for the first 12 or so years of life. Then, on a signal from the brain, the pituitary gland starts producing LH and FSH, which make the ovaries start producing several other hormones including oestrogen, progesterone and a dash of testosterone, which builds bone and muscle strength.

Oestrogen is responsible for the feminine shape – guiding the body's fat deposits into breasts, hips and thighs – and for the full development of the sex organs, including the uterus. Inside the ovaries, those innumerable tiny eggs start ripening. This is when we begin the menstrual cycles that will continue until the menopause.

The menstrual cycle

Day 1 is the first day of bleeding. It follows a drop in production of both progesterone and oestrogen. That triggers the uterus to slough off its lining, the endometrium, which is not needed because conception has not taken place. Oestrogen levels are low, which allows the production of FSH to start rising. You may be able to feel the uterus contracting to push the endometrium out.

By the end of the first week, bleeding has stopped. FSH has stimulated one of the follicles to grow, and the follicle now starts producing oestrogen. This in turn reduces FSH levels during the second week, while oestrogen levels peak during the second and third weeks.

About day 14 of a 28-day cycle, LH levels rise sharply, for just long enough to trigger ovulation. The follicle expels the egg into the fallopian tube on its way to the womb. Testosterone production also soars at this time. The collapsed follicle (now called the corpus luteum) then produces progesterone during weeks 3 and 4, to prepare the womb for a pregnancy.

If the egg has not been fertilized, the cycle ends with another burst of testosterone, and a steep fall in levels of oestrogen and progesterone. This causes the womb to shed its unused lining, the endometrium, and the cycle starts again.

Pregnancy

If the egg has been fertilized, levels of oestrogen and progesterone do not drop and there's no bleeding. Instead, the developing placenta starts producing HCG: this is the hormone that pregnancy tests find in a pregnant woman's urine just days after the first missed period. HCG steps up the ovaries' production of oestrogen and progesterone; later these will be mainly produced by the placenta. Oestrogen and a natural progestogen build up the endometrium, increase blood supply to the womb and breasts and relax the muscles around the womb to make room as the baby grows.

During childbirth, other hormones come into play, including oxytocin to help the womb contract during and after labour, prolactin to stimulate milk production, and the body's natural painkillers, beta-endorphins.

After childbirth, levels of these hormones drop sharply, and the menstrual cycle starts up again.

Menopause

As you reach the end of your thirties, hormone levels start to change. Your fertility is declining, but you probably won't notice any signs until you're in your forties. The time leading up to the menopause – the final menstrual period – and just afterwards is called the perimenopause.

Progesterone levels are starting to fall at this time. Oestrogen levels may also fall, or they may remain high during the first few years but fluctuate with sharp drops and peaks.

FSH levels may also fluctuate, but are usually quite high; the same may happen with LH. This may be what causes the classic menopausal symptom, hot flushes. The egg follicles, reaching the end of their lives, are slow to react to the stimulation of FSH and LH, so the body increases its production of these hormones to try to provoke a response. Because FSH and LH are controlled by the part of the brain that regulates temperature, high levels of them are believed to make the blood vessels suddenly dilate, causing a flush of heat.

Eventually, oestrogen levels will fall so far that your periods stop: that's the menopause. After the final period, oestrogen levels continue to fall for a while, and some menopausal symptoms may continue for a few years. But eventually the hormones settle into their new routine. Oestrogen and progesterone levels remain low, FSH and LH higher than before.

All the above explains how the whole system is meant to work. And for most of us, it does work pretty well most of the time. But many elements can go slightly awry and derail this steady functioning. The next chapter looks at how things can go wrong, and what that may lead to.

3

Conditions that may lead to hysterectomy

You may have read the previous chapter, about the smooth functioning of the reproductive system, with a wry smile. As you undoubtedly know, things don't always work as they should. This chapter looks at the conditions that may lead to your doctor offering you a hysterectomy. The following chapters detail the other options available to treat each condition.

Gynaecological problems are very widespread, especially connected with the menstrual cycle. Most women at some time have felt irritable or depressed for no apparent reason just before a period starts. Premenstrual syndrome (PMS) is a very common hormonal imbalance. Period pain and heavy bleeding are widespread too. For most of us, these are minor troubles. But in some women they are severe enough to disrupt their everyday life.

It's not just a question of having a high or a low pain threshold. Doctors have started to realize that women's bodies vary greatly in their sensitivity to hormones and to hormonal changes. So some of the conditions for which hysterectomy has often been recommended, in severe cases – such as flooding, intense pain or violent PMS – are extreme forms of normal menstrual events.

Growths in the womb are also surprisingly common. Cancer, of course, must never be overlooked. But very few of these growths – such as polyps, fibroids or adenomyomas – are malignant. The questions for most of us are: Do they hurt? Are they likely to become cancerous? And will they affect fertility?

Pain is one of the main reasons women seek their doctor's advice. That is sensible, as pain can warn of numerous different conditions, some of them potentially serious. Other than dysmenorrhoea – painful periods – there are several conditions, such as endometriosis or pelvic inflammatory disease, that can cause pelvic pain. Sometimes the uterus can even slip out of place.

The following conditions (in alphabetical order) may lead to a hysterectomy. Read on to find out what causes them, what the symptoms are and whether you can consider other forms of treatment.

Adenomyosis

An adenomyoma is endometrial tissue (from the endometrium, or inner lining of the womb) growing in the myometrium, or muscle layer. The condition, called adenomyosis, often causes heavy or painful periods.

No one knows for certain what causes adenomyosis. It may result from an operation that breaks the barrier between the endometrium and myometrium, such as sterilization, Caesarean or abortion. But the same effect could be caused naturally by pregnancy. Like other growths in the uterus, it's fuelled by oestrogen, which is probably why it's most likely to happen in women in their thirties and forties, and tends to diminish after the menopause.

Adenomyomas are important to know about, because they may be an undiagnosed cause of heavy bleeding. An operation to cure heavy bleeding by removing the endometrium would not help, because it's not coming from there. This is an example of why it's important to get a correct diagnosis.

Once doctors know what they're dealing with, medical science offers milder alternatives before you need to consider a hysterectomy.

Cancer

Cancer can appear in the uterus in several places, but occurs most often in the womb lining, which is why the term 'uterine cancer' usually means endometrial cancer. However, there are less common forms of womb cancer, including adenocanthomas and sarcomas. Leiomyosarcoma, or cancer of the muscle wall, is the most common of these.

Cancer can also develop in the neck of the womb (cervical cancer), ovary (ovarian cancer) or, less commonly, in the fallopian tubes.

Because cancer is life-threatening, if a hysterectomy is recommended it should be done *as soon as possible*. In some cases, smaller operations are possible. Chemotherapy (drug treatment) and radiotherapy may also be necessary. And there is a wealth of complementary and self-help therapies available as a back-up to orthodox treatment.

Cervical cancer

Unlike ovarian and endometrial cancer, cervical cancer is more common in young women. It usually develops from a sexually transmitted infection called human papillomavirus (HPV). You're more at risk the earlier you had your first sexual experience, the more sexual partners you've had, if you've had seven or more children, if you've been on the Pill more than five years and if you smoke. Barrier methods of contraception such as the diaphragm or condoms may reduce the risk, but this is not known for certain.

Symptoms include bleeding between periods, after sex or after the menopause, periods becoming longer and heavier, pelvic pain or painful sex.

A smear (Pap) test should pick up early signs of cervical cancer, or pre-cancerous changes called cervical dysplasia. Every woman should have a smear test at least once every three years throughout her adult life. In this very brief procedure, which should be painless, a slender instrument is inserted into your vagina to take a tiny sample from the mouth of your womb. Detecting changes allows treatment in time to prevent cancer taking hold.

Thanks to the widespread use of the smear test, cervical cancer is now usually discovered early enough for treatment to have a very good chance of success. Depending on the size of the tumour, you may be offered surgery, radiotherapy, chemotherapy or more than one of these. If you need surgery but still hope to have children, and your cancer is at an early enough stage, you may be able to have an operation called a radical trachelectomy, which preserves most of your uterus. However, as with any test, no technique is 100 per cent guaranteed. So never ignore new symptoms, especially if they include pain or bleeding.

Cancer of the womb lining (endometrial cancer)

The longer you've been exposed to oestrogen, the higher your risk of endometrial cancer: if you started your periods early or reached menopause later than average, or if you've never had a baby (as oestrogen levels are lower throughout pregnancy). If you're using HRT or taking oestrogen in any other form, you need to take a progestogen to prevent the oestrogen causing endometrial cancer.

Having a hormonal disorder called polycystic ovary syndrome (PCOS) increases your risk of developing endometrial cancer, because it suppresses ovulation. The breast cancer drug tamoxifen can also increase the risk of endometrial cancer, so you should have a pelvic check-up at least once a year if you are taking this medicine.

Endometrial cancer is also more likely to develop if you're past the menopause, overweight or white. You're at lower risk if you're slim, black, young and physically active; if you've taken the combined contraceptive Pill; and if you eat a low-fat diet. The more babies you've had, and the longer you breastfed, the lower your risk of endometrial cancer.

Cancer of the womb lining will not show up on a smear test. Symptoms include bleeding between periods or after sex; pelvic pain; painful sex or urination; or unusual vaginal discharge. These are more likely to be symptoms of other gynaecological conditions, but just in case it's cancer they should always be reported to your doctor. Investigations will include taking a biopsy, or tissue sample, from inside your womb.

Cancer of the ovary

Symptoms of ovarian cancer include pressure or pain in the pelvis, abdomen, back or legs; digestive upsets such as nausea, flatulence, constipation or diarrhoea; abdominal bloating; and exhaustion. Less common symptoms are shortness of breath, frequency of urination, or non-menstrual bleeding.

You're more at risk of ovarian cancer if you're overweight or have used fertility drugs (especially if you did not become pregnant). There's a genetic element, so be especially alert to any signs if ovarian cancer has affected your mother or sister, or two other close relatives such as aunts. And it has been suggested that using talcum powder on the perineum (the area between the vagina and anus) may increase the risk.

Your risk is lowered if you have used hormonal contraception (such as the Pill), given birth to at least one baby, breastfed, been sterilized or had a hysterectomy.

When you go to your doctor for a diagnosis, you'll probably be given a pelvic examination, blood tests and an ultrasound. You may then need an operation – either open abdominal surgery or a laparoscopy – so a surgeon can take a look at your ovaries. Small cysts can be removed at the same time. If cancer is found, you'll probably be offered a removal of the ovaries, and often a hysterectomy as well. You may be offered chemotherapy too.

If you still hope to have children and the cancer is found at an early enough stage, you may be able to keep your uterus and have just the one affected ovary removed, with chemotherapy afterwards.

Dysmenorrhoea (painful periods)

There are two kinds of dysmenorrhoea, and it's important to know which you have in order to receive the right treatment.

Primary (or spasmodic) dysmenorrhoea is period pain that's not caused by any other gynaecological condition. Anything up to half the female population suffers from this, in some cases badly enough to seek medical help. It usually occurs during the first three days of a period.

The younger you were when your periods started, the more likely you are to suffer primary dysmenorrhoea. It is also more common among smokers and women who haven't had children. And if you've had it since your teens without much change, it's also more likely to be primary.

About one sufferer in ten has what's called secondary (or congestive) dysmenorrhoea. In this case, period pain is being exacerbated by another condition, such as endometriosis or fibroids. The pain may start during the few days before you bleed, and you may also suffer from painful sex. It's especially important to get a diagnosis if your painful periods could be secondary dysmenorrhoea. It could be a warning of a gynaecological condition that can be cured if treated early enough.

Orthodox medicines and self-help can ease primary dysmenorrhoea. Secondary dysmenorrhoea should respond to treatment for the condition that's causing it.

Endometrial hyperplasia

This excessive growth of the womb lining is dangerous, as it often leads on to endometrial cancer. It's one of the possible causes of heavy or abnormal bleeding, which is why it's important to get a diagnosis if you are bleeding more than usual or have any other related concerns – even just a gut instinct that something is wrong.

It's caused by oestrogen, or by a shortage of the counteracting hormone progesterone. That's why the first forms of hormone replacement therapy (HRT), which used oestrogen alone, caused the death of many women from endometrial cancer. But it isn't restricted to women who have taken oestrogen in any form. Women who have never touched the contraceptive Pill or HRT can develop endometrial hyperplasia, and go on to get cancer.

Later chapters detail self-help measures that may reduce the risk of a recurrence. As with cancer, however, if you've already got it, this isn't a time to try self-help or alternative therapies. You won't necessarily need a hysterectomy, as doctors have some less invasive options. But don't delay in starting treatment, as it could save your life.

Endometriosis

This is another condition, like adenomyosis, in which tissue from the endometrium grows in the wrong place. In endometriosis, it grows outside the uterus, and can spread widely enough to cause bands of scar-like tissue called adhesions around other organs. It is believed to be caused by 'retrograde menstruation'. This means that when the womb lining is sloughed off during a period, some of it gets into the fallopian tubes and is carried into the pelvis, instead of going out through the cervix and leaving the body.

The main symptom of endometriosis is pain – painful sex, painful periods, painful urination or bowel movement, or just constant or intermittent pelvic pain. The more it spreads, the more damage it causes to other internal organs. It can disrupt the menstrual cycle and even mimic the symptoms of irritable bowel syndrome (IBS). It has the potential to become serious, creating cysts that can rupture and need emergency surgery. It can also cause a life-threatening ectopic pregnancy, when the fertilized egg is implanted outside the womb. Endometriosis is also a common cause of infertility and has been linked with certain cancers.

Although it can develop at any time of life, endometriosis is oestrogen-dependent and therefore is most common during the twenties to forties. It runs in families, to some extent. Other than that, its cause is uncertain.

This is one condition for which even old-time doctors may be reluctant to carry out a hysterectomy, as that sometimes causes endometriosis to spread. There are less invasive treatments, and many women try complementary therapies too.

Fibroids

These growths of smooth muscle and fibrous tissue can develop anywhere in the pelvic region, but are most often found on the inside wall of the uterus. They're sometimes also known as fibromas, fibromyomas, leiomyomas or myomas. Depending on where they grow, fibroids are described as:

- submucosal or submucous, meaning they have grown just under the womb lining;
- intramural (by far the commonest), developing between the muscles in the wall of the uterus;
- subserosal, outside the uterus; or
- pedunculated, growing on a stem from inside the womb to outside.

Fibroids can grow to the size of a melon, though the problems they cause are not related to their size. Their common symptoms are painful or heavy periods, bleeding between periods, painful sex, an uncomfortable feeling of pressure in the pelvis or a need to urinate frequently.

Fibroids may reduce your chance of becoming pregnant, especially if they are submucosal. Some research suggests that women with fibroids are as likely to become pregnant as anyone else. But if you want to have a baby, it's not just about conceiving but about having a successful pregnancy. Fibroids are thought to cause miscarriage or premature birth. So if you're having difficulty either becoming or staying pregnant, it is worth asking a specialist for advice about your fibroids, specifically in relation to your fertility problems.

Using ultrasound, doctors have recently discovered that fibroids are far more common than we used to think. Some researchers estimate that by the age of 50, about three-quarters of women are likely to have at least one. But the majority are painless, so they're unlikely to be discovered if you never have an ultrasound. They don't tend to become cancerous, so they're only worth removing if they're bothering you. Most fibroids stop causing problems after the menopause.

You're more likely to have them if other women in your family do too – but as most fibroids don't cause any trouble, and they were hard to spot before the use of ultrasound, you may not know your family history. You're at a much higher risk of having fibroids, and at an earlier age, if you're black. They're also more likely in childless women and those who are overweight, drink much alcohol or have high blood pressure.

Fibroids have been one of the commonest reasons for hysterectomy in the past. Today, medical science has far more to offer, in treatments that, unlike hysterectomy, may not end your ability to have children and could even improve it if fibroids were causing infertility. Complementary therapies and self-help techniques can also help with fibroids.

Heavy menstrual bleeding (menorrhagia, or dysfunctional uterine bleeding: DUB)

This is officially defined as a loss of more than 80ml of blood in one period, about half a teacupful. But that's very hard to measure, not only because it's usually soaked up by pads or tampons. The 'blood' you lose each month is largely tissue from the womb lining; hospital laboratories are able to calculate the amount of blood it contains. Some estimates show that many women lose more than this amount of blood without any problem. Others feel drained by a smaller blood loss.

So more useful criteria are that your periods continue for a week or more in full flow; you're losing enough to make you feel unwell; or you're passing blood clots. (The blood starts to clot when you run out of the anti-clotting chemical produced by the body to help slough off the womb lining.)

The most important factor, and the reason to seek treatment, is the impact your bleeding is having on you. Women usually go to their doctors because they are either feeling weakened by the amount of blood they're losing, or constantly flooding, or also suffering from painful cramping and backache.

The psychological effects of flooding should not be overlooked. The distress caused by soaking through the thickest pads can make some women unwilling to leave the house. And routine use of the highest-absorbency tampons has been associated with a dangerous condition called toxic-shock syndrome.

In addition, heavy periods reduce your body's stock of iron, which in itself is enough to leave you feeling unwell throughout the month. If untreated, this leads to anaemia, an iron-deficiency condition that can become serious. It's easily treated with iron supplements, but these can cause certain problems themselves, so they must only be taken on a doctor's advice and after a blood test has shown that you are lacking iron.

Heavy bleeding is common, especially in the last few years before the menopause when hormones become unbalanced. But that doesn't mean that there's no need to have an accurate diagnosis. There are many possible causes for heavy bleeding, so do persist in asking for a diagnostic procedure such as ultrasound if the simplest hormone treatments don't work or you have any other concern. It can be caused by hormones alone, or be a side effect of many pelvic disorders including fibroids, adenomyomas, endometrial hyperplasia or sometimes even cancer. Some of these are dangerous and need prompt treatment.

Some women who lose a lot of blood each month turn out to have a bleeding disorder. This can be treated too, and may mean you don't need surgery. Do you bruise easily or have nosebleeds? Do you lose a lot of blood after minor operations such as having a tooth out, or during childbirth? Has anyone in your family got a bleeding disorder? These are clues that your heavy blood loss may be caused by something other than hormones.

You'd probably know if there was haemophilia in your family, as your male relatives would be badly affected. But there are lesser-known conditions that also make you bleed excessively. The most common, found in up to 20 per cent of women with menorrhagia who were tested for it, is von Willebrands disease. This is diagnosed by a blood test for shortage of a protein that helps blood clot, von Willebrands factor. The condition is usually hereditary, but occasionally develops later in life as a result of certain health conditions, including an underactive thyroid. There are drugs you can take for it, so if your heavy bleeding can't be controlled by other methods it may be worth following this up.

Heavy blood loss can also be a side effect of some other conditions described in this chapter, in which case they need to be diagnosed and treated too.

Abnormal bleeding or discharge

The 'heavy bleeding' covered by this book means heavy blood loss during a period. Bleeding at other times is not normal and should always be investigated. Go to your doctor if you notice any bleeding, whether painful or not, when it is:

- between periods (especially if you are over 40);
- after intercourse; or
- after the menopause.

Any non-menstrual bleeding may be an early sign of a condition that needs prompt treatment. Using HRT can sometimes cause bleeding after the menopause, but don't take this for granted – get it checked by your doctor.

The same applies if you have a discharge that's unusual for you, especially if:

- it's a thin or clear discharge; and
- you have passed the menopause.

Menorrhagia is the commonest cause for hysterectomy, and yet there are many medical and surgical options you can consider first; see the following chapters.

Pelvic inflammatory disease (PID)

Bacterial infections can enter a woman's pelvis in a number of ways, but the most usual is through the vagina into the uterus. As the cervix is normally a barrier to infection, bacteria can be let in by anything that pushes through it – during childbirth or an abortion, or even having an intrauterine contraceptive device (IUD) installed. There's a possibility that making love during a period raises the risk, as the cervix is open at this time to expel the womb lining.

PID is sometimes a result of a sexually transmitted disease such as gonorrhoea or chlamydia, so you should ask to be tested for those. It's more common the more sexual partners you have, but you can reduce the risk to some degree by using barrier contraception – male or female condoms, a cap or diaphragm with spermicide. There's a possibility that douching – washing inside the vagina with chemical solutions – increases the risk of PID; douching is not a good idea anyway, as it disrupts the body's self-cleaning processes and increases the risk of skin reactions.

PID can cause excruciating period pains, along with lower back pain, sharp pains during or after sex and a dull ache in the abdomen that may spread down the thighs. Other symptoms may include fever, chills, nausea, pain when urinating, an unpleasant vaginal discharge or bleeding between periods.

These distressing symptoms should alert you to the fact that something is wrong and are a strong motivation to get to the doctor, or genitourinary medicine (GUM) clinic, at once. PID needs prompt treatment because it has bad long-term effects. The infection can move up into the fallopian tubes, causing an inflammatory condition called salpingitis in which the walls swell so that the eggs can't go through to the uterus.

Unfortunately, some women never notice any symptoms, or take them for normal period pains. This can result in long-term damage to the area, with an increased risk of infertility and ectopic pregnancy: a dangerous condition in which the embryo grows outside the womb.

PID can be cleared up if it's diagnosed quickly enough, so a hysterectomy should only be suggested if all else has failed.

Polyps

Polyps are little growths inside the womb, something like the skin tags that often develop on ageing skin. They can happen at any time of life, and may cause irregular bleeding. More importantly, though harmless at first they occasionally go on to become cancerous. And they need to be checked out because they can't always be distinguished from cancerous growths.

Polyps are quite common, and often cause irregular bleeding – it can be a relief when they're diagnosed, as many other reasons for bleeding between periods are more serious. However, they're a bit difficult to diagnose, as even an ultrasound can't always pick them up clearly. It may be necessary for your doctor to take a biopsy, which is quite similar to the cervical smear we're advised to have regularly. The instrument goes in a little further and the doctor removes a tiny amount of tissue from inside the uterus via the vagina. If you have abnormal bleeding and have been told it's caused by polyps, you do need to be sure it has been correctly diagnosed.

Like fibroids, polyps can become 'pedunculated', or growing on a stalk. If this extends through the cervix into the vagina, it can cause pain.

If you're not getting any symptoms from your polyps, you may prefer to do nothing and have your doctor keep an eye on them for any changes over the years. Otherwise, they can be removed by minor procedures, without having a hysterectomy.

Premenstrual syndrome (PMS)

This very common hormonal imbalance usually strikes during the few days before a period starts. Its symptoms, once blamed on oestrogen alone, are now thought to be sometimes caused by an abnormal response to changing levels of hormones, particularly progesterone.

PMS takes different forms, but most women with PMS will have several of the following: fluid retention (bloating), breast tenderness, headaches, exhaustion, irritability, mood swings, depression, panic attacks, inability to concentrate, food cravings. Most women who have it find that they get either the aggressive symptoms, or the depressive symptoms, with or without the physical effects. About one woman in 20 has it badly enough to need treatment. And when it's severe it can make women violent: it's even been used as a defence in court cases.

One sign that it's PMS rather than anything else is that it normally stops as soon as a period starts. And in most women it lasts just a couple of days. But in some women, the symptoms can affect them for anything up to the last two weeks of the cycle. If left untreated, it tends to get worse as you grow older – until, of course, it is ended by the menopause.

Luckily, it's one of the easiest gynaecological conditions to treat with self-help measures, including dietary changes. Doctors, too, have effective alternatives to offer. Hysterectomy would rarely be carried out these days for PMS alone.

Uterine prolapse

In later age or after many pregnancies, the uterus may sag into the vagina. It happens when the pelvic-floor muscles are weak and the womb's supporting ligaments have been stretched too much. When people mention a 'prolapse', they usually mean this kind. It is the reason for about half of all hysterectomies undergone by women over 50 and of about one in eight of all hysterectomies in the UK.

Your uterus is more likely to prolapse if you are heavily overweight, suffer from a chronic cough or constipation, have large fibroids or other uterine growths, or do work that involves heavy lifting. It's also more common if you're white than if you're black or Asian. Uterine prolapse doesn't always cause problems, and some women don't even know it's happened. But it may cause pain in the vagina and lower back, a 'dragging' feeling or sense of pressure, painful sex and problems with pregnancy. Symptoms often ease off when you're lying down.

Treatment for a prolapsed womb depends on how weak the supporting muscles and ligaments have become. There are medical and surgical alternatives to hysterectomy, as well as self-help.

Other organs in the pelvic area can also prolapse, including the rectum (a condition called a rectocele), the small intestine (enterocele), bladder (cystocele), urethra (urethrocele), or both the bladder and urethra (cystourethrocele). These would not be treated by hysterectomy. However, they can cause problems by pressing on the vagina, and may complicate the diagnosis of uterine prolapse. One prolapsed organ can push others out of place if not treated in time.

4

Finding out what's wrong

One of the reasons women used to be hurried into having a hysterectomy is that conditions were often not diagnosed until a late stage. By that time there may have been few other options. Now, not only are there many more ways of treating gynaecological conditions, there are more and better ways of making a correct diagnosis. Many conditions can now be identified early enough for treatment with self-help therapies and gentle medicines. So don't soldier on when you're in pain or half-fainting with blood loss. Go to the doctor while you are still well enough to take the time non-surgical options may need.

The first and vital step towards recovery is to get a diagnosis of anything that's bothering you. A large number of gynaecological conditions have overlapping symptoms, such as pelvic pain, heavy blood loss or abdominal swelling. You need to ensure that you're being treated for the right cause. It can take time to disentangle the symptoms and identify exactly what's giving rise to them.

Is infertility your main concern?

If you are trying unsuccessfully for a baby and have one of the conditions in this book, don't presume that it is the cause of your infertility. It's true that some of these conditions may reduce the chance of a successful pregnancy. But it is common to be able to give birth despite having endometriosis, fibroids or other growths.

Many women only have these removed in the hopes of becoming pregnant. However, treatments for gynaecological conditions may reduce your chances still further, even if they aim to leave the uterus undamaged.

Your lack of success so far may have another cause that needs to be diagnosed. So do push to find out exactly why you are not conceiving. Discuss your hopes with your doctor before agreeing to any treatment, especially surgery.

Making a diagnosis

A doctor's first line of enquiry is to ask you, the patient, about your symptoms. For this reason, it's a good idea to jot down some notes to remind you to mention everything that seems relevant. If you are asked further questions that don't seem to have any bearing on your symptoms, this is usually in order to exclude other conditions that have some of the same kind of symptoms.

An internal examination is usually done next, via your vagina, as when you're having a smear test. Blood and urine tests can reveal whether you're lacking anything your body needs – iron as a result of heavy bleeding, for example – or making too much or too little of any of the hormones that keep the system functioning, or fighting an infection.

Sometimes doctors take a sample for analysis. This may be as quick and painless as a swab, when they simply wipe some secretions, for example from your vagina, onto a cotton-wool bud. Or they may need to take a biopsy – a small amount of tissue – from inside the uterus for analysis. This can be done by endometrial aspiration, in which a narrow tube is passed along the vagina into your womb and some endometrial cells are removed by suction. In dilation and curettage (D&C), a small sample is scraped out of the uterus. However, neither of these allows the doctor to see inside.

Advances in medical science have made many conditions easier to diagnose as well as to treat. Specifically, a range of non-invasive techniques are now used to create a visible picture of what's inside the body. These allow doctors to see changes inside our bodies that once could only have been guessed at, or inferred through the use of medical detective work.

Ultrasound – the use of sound waves – is the one most people know best, for providing parents-to-be with their first pictures of the baby inside the womb. It is also a useful diagnostic tool. A painless scanner is moved over your abdomen, while the changing picture shows on a screen.

To aid diagnosis of a condition inside your womb, you may also be offered a trans-vaginal scan, in which a much smaller scanner, about the size of a tampon, is inserted into your vagina. A further refinement, called sonohysterography, involves having a harmless sterile saline solution inserted into your uterus before the trans-vaginal scan. The fluid gives much better visibility, especially showing the contrast between normal and abnormal tissue.

X-rays have been in use for many decades, but are limited in what they can show; there's also a health risk in having too much electromagnetic radiation. Computed tomography (CAT) scans take X-rays from a number of angles to build up a more detailed image. Magnetic resonance imaging (MRI) uses magnets and radio waves. CAT scans and MRIs can feel a bit intimidating or claustrophobic, as you're surrounded by machinery.

Some valuable diagnostic procedures are slightly more invasive, but useful in giving a clear view of what's inside. A hysteroscope is a camera on a thin tube that's inserted into your uterus through the vagina. This useful little device can show the entire uterus and the fallopian tubes, and have instruments passed down inside it to carry out minor operations such as removing polyps or taking a biopsy. A laparoscopy involves the doctor making a small incision in your abdomen and inserting a thin tube with a light on the end of it. The laparoscope can be used to show the outside as well as the inside of the uterus.

Any of the procedures described can help the doctor to build up a picture of what's causing your symptoms. As the same symptoms can have several causes, it's essential to get the diagnosis right. Prescribing drugs to control heavy bleeding, for example, could be ineffective if it's caused by fibroids, and a waste of potentially life-saving time if it's caused by cancer.

Don't ignore pain or exhaustion

Pelvic pain should always be investigated, especially if you're feeling it between periods or after the menopause. It can be a sign of many gynaecological conditions, or of other diseases. Don't accept pain relief without a diagnosis, because pain is often a warning of something that needs treatment.

Similarly, unexplained exhaustion is often a sign of ill-health. You may have come to think of it as a natural part of a busy life, especially when you are also coping with a gynaecological condition. But it should not be.

The first thing to do, if you are always tired, is to slow down a little and try to offload some of your work. Get a few early nights and take some time off. But if those simple remedies don't work, speak to your doctor, who can test you for common conditions that can drain a woman's energy.

5

What are the options for my condition?

The belief that hysterectomy solves most gynaecological problems is dying out as doctors become familiar with new treatments. Some still have more confidence in what they see as a tried-and-tested cure, yet hysterectomies aren't a cure-all and may cause problems in their turn (see Chapter 9 for arguments for and against).

Cancer and pre-cancerous conditions such as endometrial hyperplasia should always be treated as a matter of urgency. But certain other cases don't need any treatment at all, and some need to be weighed up very carefully. Surgery aimed at cutting out endometriosis, for example, sometimes has the effect of spreading it more widely.

As shown in Chapter 3, hysterectomy is a possible treatment for many conditions. But except in the case of cancers, it's worth considering all other options first. The next chapters explain what each one entails.

Like anyone else, doctors can become set in their ways. Also, surgeons tend to be most proficient at the operation they carry out most often. It's natural that they prefer to do what they do best, for the sake of their patients. But if, after hearing your own consultant's advice, you still wish to try a different option, you can ask to be referred to someone who specializes in that area.

Note: The self-help measures detailed in Chapters 12 to 15 can be used at the same time as the medical or surgical alternatives described in Chapters 6 and 7, unless clearly stated otherwise, because they don't clash. Complementary and alternative (CAM) therapies, however, may not work in combination with orthodox treatments, so look at Chapter 8 to check on this.

Adenomyosis

Painkilling non-steroidal anti-inflammatory drugs (NSAIDs) and hormonal drugs are the main non-surgical treatments for adenomyosis. These can relieve the symptoms but don't cure the growths.

Unfortunately, surgery such as endometrial ablation is rarely suitable, as it only removes the lining of the womb, not the tissue that has grown into the underlying muscle.

It may be a question of weighing up your present symptoms against the results of having a hysterectomy.

See later chapters on medical options, hysterectomy, self-help, stress relief and nutrition.

Cancer

Survival rates for cancer are improving all the time. Hysterectomy is the standard treatment for cancers of the reproductive system, and is often enough to cure the disease by itself. Otherwise, you may need radiotherapy or chemotherapy.

If you have a cancer of the uterus – the most likely is endometrial cancer – you will probably be offered a radical hysterectomy. A hysterectomy is also usual when cancer is found in the cervix. However, in some cases of cervical cancer, a radical trachelectomy may be possible instead. If it is in an ovary, you may need as little removed as the one ovary, or as much as a radical hysterectomy.

See later chapters on medical options, surgical options, CAM, hysterectomy, self-help, stress relief, exercise and nutrition.

Dysmenorrhoea

If your doctor suspects your period pains may be secondary dysmenorrhoea, diagnosis will include a number of tests to identify the underlying cause. That can then be treated.

Much can be done to ease primary dysmenorrhoea. First, you're likely to be offered painkilling NSAIDs, the contraceptive Pill or a Mirena coil. If these don't help, you may be offered the antiprogestogen drug danazol. Surgeons used to offer a nerve-cutting operation called uterine nerve ablation, but this has not been found effective in the long term.

See later chapters on medical options, surgical options, CAM, self-help, stress relief, exercise and nutrition.

Endometrial hyperplasia

This is one of the conditions that must be treated as soon as possible, because it can often develop into endometrial cancer.

The first treatment is likely to be high-dose progestogens, either as tablets or in the Mirena intrauterine system. If this doesn't make enough difference, you may be offered endometrial ablation, which should solve the problem as it destroys the uterine lining. However, endometrial ablation is often only partially successful and needs to be repeated. It is important to ensure that your uterine lining has been completely removed, even if it takes more than one operation.

See later chapters on medical options, surgical options, self-help and nutrition.

Endometriosis

The first line of treatment is with NSAIDS, such as ibuprofen and naproxen. These fight the inflammation caused by endometriosis, as well as relieving pain. If you don't get on with NSAIDS, you could try paracetamol, which is less powerful but has few side effects as long as you are very careful not to take more than the stated dose.

The next stage is hormonal drugs, to counteract the body's production of oestrogen. These could be the combined contraceptive Pill, progestogens, antiprogestogens or GnRH agonists (see page 8).

Surgery can remove much of the endometrial tissue that has grown outside the womb. This is usually done with lasers, but some doctors now believe excision – cutting it out – is more effective. The operation is usually done by 'keyhole' surgery, through a small incision near your navel. If the endometriosis is very widespread, you may need open abdominal surgery. Although the operation relieves symptoms for some time, endometriosis can keep growing back until you reach the menopause.

It is possible to cut the nerves carrying pain signals between the brain and the uterus, but this hasn't been proved effective enough to be widely carried out.

Hysterectomy should be avoided if possible, as it can have the accidental effect of spreading endometriosis.

See later chapters on medical options, surgical options, CAM, self-help, stress-relief, exercise and nutrition.

Fibroids

There are two reasons for having fibroids treated: either because they are causing painful symptoms or because they are preventing you carrying a pregnancy to term. However, some of the most effective treatments put an end to child-bearing. So you need to check with your doctor from the start that you are not doing anything that would reduce your chance of a successful pregnancy still further.

The first line of treatment is usually hormonal: the combined contraceptive Pill, the Mirena coil or drugs such as GnRH agonists. These have short-term effects, and can be used to shrink fibroids to an easier size for removal. This treatment may be suitable if you want to have children, as the size of fibroids may be reduced for long enough for you to get pregnant and have a baby. Check with your doctor if this would be appropriate in your case.

The long-term treatments are surgical. Uterine artery embolization (UAE) and myomectomy are both intended to destroy fibroids while protecting the uterus and maintaining fertility, though this cannot be guaranteed. Myolysis is another possibility, but future fertility is less certain. Endometrial ablation is minimally invasive, and certain methods can remove fibroids. However, you cannot have children after endometrial ablation. New ultrasound and laser treatments have not yet been in use long enough to recommend.

Operations to remove fibroids often have to be repeated, sometimes more than once. Up to now, quite a few women have gone on to have hysterectomies anyway. But as the alternative treatments become more widely practised and more advanced, the long-term success rate is improving.

Heavy menstrual bleeding (menorrhagia)

In the early 1990s, about two-thirds of women who went to their doctor about heavy bleeding ended up having a hysterectomy. This has changed enormously. The first step is to ensure that your bleeding is purely part of your menstrual cycle, and not caused by anything that needs immediate treatment, such as cancer, or that could be differently treated, such as fibroids.

The current standard procedure for menorrhagia, recommended by the UK National Institute for Health and Clinical Excellence (NICE) in 2007, is to start by trying the Mirena intrauterine system (IUS), which releases progestogen. This is suitable if you're willing to have a device inserted and prepared to stay with it for a year or so, giving any initial problems time to settle down. If you don't want to use an IUS, you're likely to be offered either a combined contraceptive Pill, NSAIDs, or (if you don't need pain relief) tranexamic acid. If these aren't suitable, the next choice is norethisterone tablets, or possibly three-monthly progestogen injections.

If these don't help, and you don't want any further pregnancies, you may be offered endometrial ablation. NICE recommends second-generation techniques where possible: impedance-controlled bipolar radiofrequency ablation, thermal balloon ablation, microwave ablation or free-fluid thermal ablation (see Chapter 7).

Not every doctor agrees with these guidelines. Some, for example, have said this understates the Mirena's possible side effects. Other research, including some published by independent reviewers the Cochrane Collaboration, suggests that first-generation endometrial ablation techniques are less likely to cause perforation of the uterus, because the surgeon can see better through the hysteroscope.

If none of these works, and there's nothing, such as hidden fibroids, that could be making you bleed excessively, you may wish to consider a hysterectomy.

If your heavy bleeding is caused by fibroids, see that section (above) for the next steps.

See later chapters on medical options, surgical options, CAM, self-help, stress relief and nutrition.

Pelvic inflammatory disease (PID)

Once PID has been diagnosed you should be prescribed antibiotics. This should be done as soon as possible, because PID can cause long-term damage, including infertility.

As it is sometimes caused by a sexually transmitted infection (STI), you and your partner should both be tested and treated if necessary. If you do need treatment, you'll be advised not to have unprotected sex until that infection and the PID have cleared up. If you have a coil or intrauterine device (IUD) this should be removed. Ask your doctor whether you need emergency contraception.

If the PID persists, you may need to go to hospital to have a series of antibiotic injections. You may also need laparoscopic investigations to see if there is anything else happening inside: for example, PID can cause painful abscesses which need to be drained.

Hysterectomy should not be necessary unless long-untreated inflammation has caused severe internal damage.

See later chapters on medical options, CAM, self-help and nutrition.

Polyps

You may be offered surgery as a first step with polyps. That's because removing them also provides tissue for analysis, to check they're not malignant. They can be scraped out quite easily under general anaesthetic. Those near the cervix can usually be removed through the vagina, but larger ones and those higher up in the uterus may need to be taken out through the abdomen.

See later chapters on surgical options, stress relief and nutrition.

Premenstrual syndrome (PMS)

Exercise, dietary changes and stress relief all play such a major role in coping with PMS that they're recommended by many orthodox specialists.

Oestrogen may be prescribed to suppress the menstrual cycle, along with a progestogen to prevent the oestrogen causing cancer. The combined contraceptive Pill isn't recommended for PMS, as the progestogen is in a form that can aggravate the symptoms. The Mirena or a Pill called Yasmin may be better sources of progestogen.

Antidepressants called selective serotonin re-uptake inhibitors (SSRIs) have been effective for some forms of PMS. In severe cases, GnRH agonists may be helpful, along with add-back HRT or tibolone to prevent osteoporosis or menopausal side effects.

See later chapters on medical options, CAM, self-help, stress relief, exercise and nutrition.

Uterine prolapse

Physiotherapy is the gentlest effective treatment for a prolapse. A specialist physio can teach you an individual programme based on pelvic-floor exercises. After that, it's up to you to continue doing the exercises regularly, and it may take some months before you notice the improvement.

HRT is sometimes able to strengthen internal muscles and relieve a mild prolapse. Otherwise, you may be offered a vaginal pessary, or a double pessary if necessary. For many women, these are enough to hold the uterus in place.

If the prolapse is very severe (for example, if the cervix can be seen or felt in the vagina near the vulva), you will probably need a surgical repair. In cases where a severe prolapse has caused ulceration, a vaginal pessary can be used for a few months, along with oestrogen cream, to heal the ulcer before an operation is carried out.

Surgical repair, or suspension, involves lifting the womb and holding it in place. This can be done by sacrohysteropexy or sacrospinous fixation. An earlier procedure called the Manchester repair or Fothergill operation is no longer widely carried out as it was often unsuccessful.

See later chapters on medical options, surgical options, self-help and exercise.

Research on the internet

The internet is crammed with health advice, much of it inaccurate. From health scares that circulate by email to websites offering fake cures for terminal diseases, it's buzzing with nonsense. And you can't check the veracity of a claim by seeing how often it comes up when you do a search: the same wrong information gets copied from one site to another until it looks like widespread knowledge.

Yet among the dross is a valuable core of information. Mainstream medical sites are generally the most reliable, with one reservation: they tend to trust drugs that have more backing from the manufacturers' public-relations department than from independent research. The term 'evidence-based medicine' only came into widespread use during the 1990s. Many widely used medical and surgical treatments have never actually been proved safe or effective in independent scientific trials.

Information about health conditions may be influenced by manufacturers, according to whether they have a treatment to sell. There are numerous drugs and other products available that are intended to relieve gynaecological symptoms. Patients' groups and websites on those subjects may be promoting such products.

Look for sites put up by universities, health departments and independent research bodies. You can search for a particular word, such as your health condition, with the search restricted to a named site, such as <http://cochrane.co.uk> for the Cochrane Collaboration of independent reviewers. Or restrict your search to sites with particular endings, for example, <.ac.uk> for British universities, or <.edu> for US universities, or <.edu.au> for Australian universities, or <.nhs.uk> for the National Health Service.

There's an abundance of websites set up by women with gynaecological conditions, Many of them include forums where you can discuss your concerns and treatment options with other women who have already been through them.

6
Medical options

If you've been offered a hysterectomy but are not sure that this is for you, the first thing to do is to check that you have time to consider other routes. If a cancer has been found, you need to have it treated as soon as possible – but even some cancers can be cured without a hysterectomy. Get a second medical opinion quickly if you're not sure your doctor is right.

For most other conditions, there are at least a few options. This chapter looks at the non-surgical options, as modern medicine has a lot to offer before you even need to start considering an operation. If your doctor isn't open to considering the possibilities, you should seek the advice of other qualified experts, and do some research of your own.

The first course of action for most hormone-related symptoms will be better known as contraceptives: the Pill or the Mirena, which releases progestogen. If those aren't suitable or don't work, you may be offered one of several other medicines, from painkillers to powerful drugs. If hormones or other drugs don't solve your problem, you can now have one of numerous operations that are less drastic than a hysterectomy. These are detailed in the next chapter.

Below are details of drugs and devices and the conditions they can be used for. They are listed, as far as possible, in the order in which you are likely to encounter them.

Watchful waiting

In many conditions, the first possibility is to do nothing. Women often discover by chance that they have fibroids or polyps, during a scan for some other reason. In the past, some doctors would recommend a hysterectomy as soon as they spotted a fibroid. But in most cases fibroids don't cause any real trouble. They're not dangerous, so there's no reason to treat them unless they are causing symptoms or you are having difficulty conceiving. If a hormone-related condition discovered in your forties isn't endangering your health, you may prefer to wait for the menopause to put a natural end to it.

So if your condition is not causing any problems, your doctor may advise doing nothing for the moment. You should return to your doctor, of course, if you start to experience pain, heavy bleeding or other disturbing symptoms.

Hormonal contraceptives

Hormone-based contraceptives can play a dual role in also treating some health conditions. The advantage of this approach is that they are simple, easy to use, very well tested over many years, and their effects are totally reversible. You can stop using them any time you like, and your fertility should be back to normal within a few months.

The Pill

The first solution you're likely to be offered for heavy or painful periods is a low-dose combined (oestrogen and progestogen) contraceptive Pill. This simple solution relieves or at least reduces period problems for about half the women who use it. So it's well worth trying as a first step. A combined Pill containing norethisterone or levonorgestrel is often helpful for endometriosis.

The Pill itself causes problems for some users. But because so many women take the Pill, there are numerous different formulations available. If the first one you try doesn't help or has side effects, you may wish to try several different brands, and adjust the dosage. Side effects of the contraceptive Pill can include breakthrough bleeding, breast tenderness, acne, migraine or mood swings. It also makes you five times likelier to suffer a blood clot, or thrombosis. You're at greatest risk during your first year on the Pill and if you are overweight. You shouldn't take the Pill if you have high blood pressure, as it increases your risk of a heart attack or stroke – especially if you're approaching the menopause, when these risks increase anyway. Smoking while you're on the Pill increases your risk of a heart attack by up to ten times.

Staying on the combined Pill for more than five years increases your risk of cervical cancer, so you should be extra careful to have regular smear tests. It also slightly increases your risk of breast cancer. However, long-term use of hormonal contraception has been found to reduce your risk of other cancers, of the ovary, endometrium and bowel.

Intrauterine system (IUS) Mirena

Another product that's better known as a contraceptive is the intra-uterine system (IUS) Mirena. It's like a contraceptive coil or intrauterine device (IUD), but unlike those it contains a progestogen – the artificial form of the hormone progesterone – called levonorgestrel.

Whereas IUDs often cause painful or heavy periods, the Mirena has the opposite effect. Thanks to the progestogen, it's very effective in reducing blood loss: some women stop having periods altogether. This is a particularly good option for women over 40 or who smoke, as they should not be using oestrogen-based contraception for health reasons. It's also worth trying if you have fibroids, especially if the main symptom is heavy bleeding. There is a chance that the fibroids may prevent the progestogen from being absorbed effectively, and you may need to persevere through some initial side effects. But as with the Pill, if it's not helping enough after about three months, you don't have to continue with it.

The Mirena may have side effects, such as abdominal pain, backache, acne, headaches or breast tenderness. But these tend to wear off after the first few months. Because it is a form of hormonal contraception, it does carry some health risks and is not suitable for women who have had cancer of the breast, womb or ovaries. And as with the IUD, there's a small risk of infection.

Other medicines

The advantage of taking drugs to relieve your symptoms is that you can stop them any time you like. Like the contraceptive options, they will not diminish your long-term fertility.

Painkillers

Pain is a symptom of many gynaecological conditions, and the cause needs to be diagnosed in order to be treated. While you're undergoing investigations or waiting for treatment, though, you may be advised to take painkillers.

Over-the-counter painkillers offer a simple self-help solution. Non-steroidal anti-inflammatory drugs (NSAIDs) such as aspirin and ibuprofen are widely bought, as are paracetamol and the opioid (opium-related) drug codeine. They've helped many women through the most painful days of a bad period, or while waiting for treatment, and are safe for occasional use that way. However, it's not a good idea to take any kind of painkiller on a more regular basis. Just because they don't need a prescription, they should not be assumed to be harmless.

A doctor may prescribe stronger pain relief, such as codeine in higher doses than you can readily buy, or another opioid called tramadol. An NSAID called mefenamic acid, also known as a prostaglandin synthetase inhibitor, may be prescribed for period problems. It has some

> ### Read the instructions!
>
> Never take more than the stated dose of a medicine. Any drug can be dangerous, or even deadly, if taken in overdose. Painkillers are the most common causes of fatal overdose, along with mind-altering drugs such as antidepressants and tranquillizers. If you're not sure how much to take, go back to your doctor or pharmacist, or ring NHS Direct.
>
> But even a prescribed dose may be too high for an individual. If you have any suspicion that the dose you've been prescribed is too strong, consult your doctor or get a second opinion. You may have more than average sensitivity to its effects.

effect on heavy bleeding as well as relieving cramps. You may find these drugs control the pain as long as you take them every day. But this can have harmful effects if you continue over the long term – especially if they include codeine or tramadol, which are addictive.

All painkillers have possible side effects. If you have any known risk of the serious ones, make sure your doctor knows this and can assess the suitability of these drugs for you. NSAIDS may cause stomach upsets, internal bleeding, dizziness and possibly fluid retention. Mefenamic acid's minor side effects include nausea and nervousness, but it may also cause heart, liver or kidney problems. Paracetamol causes few every-day problems, but is the easiest to overdose on. Codeine and tramadol can cause nausea, dry membranes, constipation, breathing difficulties and drowsiness, and should not be taken if you have liver or kidney problems. These opioid painkillers also cause constipation, which exacerbates the painful symptoms of conditions such as endometriosis.

Are over-the-counter painkillers a safe alternative?

Being an opioid drug, codeine is potentially addictive. It is sold over the counter in the UK in combination with other drugs such as paracetamol and ibuprofen. As a result, people seeking more of a codeine 'hit' have taken fatal overdoses of the drug with which it is mixed. A relatively small overdose of paracetamol can cause irreversible liver damage, and an overdose of an NSAID such as ibuprofen is likely to cause internal bleeding. Several organizations (see 'Useful addresses') have been set up by and for people trying to break their addiction to opioid painkillers.

There is also concern that one's body may become dependent on painkillers. A pain that might have worn off by itself, or been cured by other treatment, may become permanent as the body loses the ability to make its own pain-relieving chemicals. People suffering from chronic pain sometimes believe that their condition stems from taking painkillers for too long.

So it is important to ensure that your doctor knows what you're taking and how long for. In particular, your doctor should be aware if you have a lung condition such as asthma, or any risk of liver or kidney problems – for example because other members of your family have them.

Drugs affecting blood flow

Tranexamic acid is an antifibrinolytic drug – one that helps blood to clot. It has been found to reduce heavy bleeding in more than half the women who use it. Although side effects aren't common, it may increase your risk of a thrombosis – a dangerous blood clot blocking a vein. If your heavy bleeding is caused by fibroids, there is also a chance that they could be damaged by the drug, causing further pain and fever. Tranexamic acid doesn't relieve pain.

Etamsylate, another drug that reduces blood flow, is sometimes used. However, NICE recommends that it should not be prescribed for heavy bleeding.

Non-contraceptive hormonal drugs

Most gynaecological conditions have a hormonal element, so hormones can play a valuable part in their treatment. The tried-and-tested contraceptive Pill and the Mirena intrauterine system are first in line for certain conditions, but others call for different hormonal options.

Oestrogen

This is more often the cause of the conditions covered in this book rather than the cure. But in the case of premenstrual syndrome (PMS) it can be a valuable treatment. PMS tends to occur either when the body is making too much of the opposing hormones, such as progesterone and androgens, or because of a woman's individual sensitivity to hormone changes.

The oestrogen component of hormone replacement therapy (HRT) is also valuable in treating mild cases of uterine prolapse, helping to rebuild and strengthen the pelvic floor.

GnRH agonists

By blocking the body's production of oestrogen, GnRH agonists can shrink fibroids, ease menorrhagia, relieve heavy bleeding and reduce the spread of endometriosis and adenomyosis. They tend to have names ending in '-relin', such as buserelin, goserelin, leuprorelin, nafarelin and triptorelin.

They are usually prescribed for a short time, to give you some relief of symptoms before the problem-causing tissue starts growing again. This can be helpful to tide you over if you're approaching the menopause, when these problems should be relieved naturally as your body's oestrogen levels fall. GnRH agonists are also useful when taken for a few months before an operation for fibroids. They reduce the size of the growths, making them easier to remove.

These drugs are not usually used before an operation for endometriosis, as that could make it harder for the surgeon to find and remove the tissue. But used for six months afterwards, they have been found to relieve pain and delay any recurrence of endometriosis.

GnRH agonists can be very effective over a few months, but should not be continued for more than six months as they mimic the effects of menopause, and can cause reduction in bone density, which leads to osteoporosis in the long term. This effect may be reduced by taking them along with HRT or the similar drug tibolone, in very low doses, known as 'add-back therapy'.

Some doctors are reluctant to prescribe GnRH agonists such as leuprorelin because of the unwanted side effects, which are similar to those of the menopause, including hot flushes, and your periods are likely to stop. You should use barrier methods of contraception while you're taking a GnRH agonist. The Pill would interact badly with it, but it is important not to get pregnant as the drug could cause miscarriage or birth defects.

Progestogens

Progestogens, such as norethisterone, are synthetic versions of the body's natural hormones. They are also known as progestins. These drugs can reduce heavy bleeding caused by fibroids, although they do not shrink the fibroids themselves. They may also be prescribed alongside GnRH agonists, to reduce the side effects and make it safe for you to take the GnRH agonists for a longer time.

Antiprogestogens

Antiprogestogens, such as danazol and gestrinone, are also known as antiprogestins or testosterone derivatives. Reducing the body's production of oestrogen and progesterone, they can ease the symptoms of endometriosis and reduce fibroid size. An antiprogestogen called mifepristone, developed as an abortion pill, has also been found to reduce the size of fibroids.

However, antiprogestogens have many side effects, such as development of masculine traits (voice deepening, facial hair) and menopausal symptoms. NICE recommends that danazol should not be prescribed for heavy bleeding.

You'll probably be asked to have a pregnancy test before you start these drugs, as they can cause birth defects. You should use non-hormonal contraception such as the diaphragm, cervical cap or condoms while you are taking these medicines.

Cancer treatments

The standard procedure for cancers of the reproductive organs is surgery to remove the organ. As a back-up, you may need to have radiotherapy: treatment with radiation to kill any remaining cancer cells. Your specialist may also prescribe hormones to block the action of your body's own hormones in fuelling the cancer. Or you may be given drugs (chemotherapy) that will either kill the cancer cells or stop them dividing.

Antibiotics

These workhorses of the medical world have a role to play in gynaecology too. They are the standard treatment for pelvic inflammatory disease (PID).

Until the middle of the twentieth century, medicine had very few weapons to fight bacterial infections, which wiped out whole populations during frequent epidemics. The discovery of antibiotics changed the face of medical practice. Antibiotics are almost miraculously effective in fighting bacteria, and have single-handedly reduced the death rate in the developed world from such one-time killers as childbirth, tuberculosis and chest infections.

Unfortunately, their success has led to so much overuse that bacteria have developed a resistance to them. So, certain infections may not respond at once to a course of antibiotics. You increase the risk of this if you start taking antibiotics but give up before completing the course. When PID is not treated in its early stages, it often becomes stubborn: a course of antibiotics will relieve the symptoms for a while, but the infection soon makes its presence felt again. And because PID often stems from infection with more than one bacterium, an antibiotic that's fatal to one organism may have little impact on the others.

This is why doctors in the past often recommended a hysterectomy, or removal of the fallopian tubes or ovaries, depending on where the infection had taken hold. But that is a drastic step for something that can be cleared up in time. You may just have to show more persistence than the infection. It may need a stay in hospital, and regular injections of powerful antibiotics, but you should eventually be free of PID with your reproductive organs intact.

Side effects

Every drug can cause side effects, and many of them are detailed on these pages. Sometimes the list of possible adverse effects could put you off taking a medicine. But they may be extremely rare, or only a risk if you have certain other health conditions. They are often minor nuisances that are outweighed by the benefit of the medicine.

The patient information leaflet provided with each drug should give you full details; or visit one of the reputable medical websites listed in 'Useful addresses'. Ask your doctor if you have any concerns about side effects. Do let your doctor know if you experience any, and ask about a change of prescription if they are a problem.

Vaginal pessary

Pessaries are used in cases of uterine prolapse. Unlike a pharmaceutical pessary, which you may have used in the past to treat a condition such as thrush, these are small devices like a contraceptive cap or diaphragm. They come in various shapes, sizes and materials including silicone and latex. If necessary, you can use two pessaries at the same time.

This may be all you need to support the uterus. It can also relieve the problems caused by other prolapsed organs pressing on the vagina.

You should be able to remove the vaginal pessary if it gets in the way when making love. Some women, especially those who never got on with tampons, may find this difficult. You need to be clear of any vaginal infections before inserting the pessary; and as some pessaries are made of latex you should let your doctor know if you're allergic to this material.

A pessary can cause irritations or infections in the vagina, so stay alert for signs such as discharge or strong odour. In very rare cases, use of a pessary has been associated with vaginal cancer. But these problems are less likely than the risk of damage being caused by a prolapse. As always when using a medical device, you should follow the instructions for care and cleaning, and have regular check-ups.

7

Surgical options

For most conditions, you'll probably first be offered some of the medical options – drugs or devices – detailed in the previous chapter. But there are also a number of operations now available that are less drastic than a hysterectomy.

Many of these operations have come into use during the past few years, so not all doctors are familiar with them. That's an understandable reason why a doctor would not recommend them. Another is that these cutting-edge treatments have not yet been widely enough used for researchers to be certain that they are safe and effective. But if the alternative is hysterectomy, you may well want to seek a second qualified opinion.

Depending on the condition you have, you may be offered the following:

- Dilation and curettage (D&C, or 'scrape')
- Endometrial ablation
- Laser surgery
- Myolysis
- Myomectomy
- Presacral neurectomy (PSN)
- Radical trachelectomy
- Sacrohysteropexy
- Sacrospinous fixation
- Ultrasound surgery
- Uterine artery embolization (UAE)
- Uterine nerve ablation (UNA)
- Uterosacral ligament resection.

Surgeons now have three different ways to access the uterus, though not every operation would allow a choice. Open abdominal surgery, or laparotomy – the traditional approach through an incision in the abdomen – allows the surgeon more space to see inside and to ensure everything necessary has been done. But it is a major operation, often leaving a large scar, and needs a longer recovery time than other less invasive procedures. In many cases, it's no longer necessary.

Using laparoscopy, or 'keyhole' surgery, surgeons can operate through a tiny incision, using a camera, light and instruments on slender tubes. This is suitable for many procedures, especially smaller ones, both inside and outside the uterus. The surgeon may also use instruments passed into the womb through the vagina, allowing the best possible range of space and visibility. Keyhole surgery requires much less time for recovery than the traditional route.

The least invasive method involves no incision at all, as the instruments are passed up the vagina and through the cervix. This does not allow a view of the pelvic area outside the uterus, but it can be used for many operations inside it. The surgeon may look into the uterus through a hysteroscope, or may operate without this. This is often done as day surgery and patients may be back on their feet the same day.

Most importantly, surgeons now have many new ways of treating non-urgent gynaecological conditions before considering a hysterectomy. These are listed below, in alphabetical order for ease of finding a name you may have been given by your doctor.

Note: Please don't be embarrassed to ask how a treatment may affect your sex life. Even if you're not sexually active at present, you may wish to be again in the future, no matter how old you are. Some operations, such as vaginal repair, can make intercourse difficult. A prolapse operation called colpocleisis, although not common, closes off the vagina altogether.

Dilation and curettage (D&C, or 'scrape')

This was once a common method of removing tissue from inside the uterus, either for analysis or in an attempt to reduce heavy bleeding. The surgeon scraped out some of the womb lining, using an instrument inserted via the vagina. It involved a general anaesthetic and an overnight stay in hospital. There was no way of seeing into the womb, so it was often unreliable.

There's no evidence that it was successful in treating any gynaecological condition, and it often caused internal damage. The development of more targeted procedures means a D&C alone is no longer widely considered a useful treatment. It is sometimes used in conjunction with a hysteroscope to get a sample of tissue for diagnosis.

Endometrial ablation or resection

This is not suitable if you want to have children, as it is intended to destroy the endometrium, or womb lining. If you did conceive afterwards, you would be at high risk of miscarriage or other problems. However, if you are not concerned about remaining fertile, it's an effective option for heavy bleeding. Some methods can also remove small submucosal fibroids and polyps.

A slender instrument is inserted into the uterus, and the womb lining is destroyed by one of a number of methods which include electric pulses, laser, radiofrequency waves, microwaves, freezing (cryotherapy), heated saline solution or a heated balloon. The operation is usually carried out under local anaesthetic.

About half the women who undergo this treatment stop menstruating after a successful ablation, and the rest have very light periods. However, it doesn't always work, and it's not uncommon to have it done more than once.

In earlier methods, known as the 'first generation', the surgeon operates while looking into the uterus through a hysteroscope. Some of the latest, second-generation procedures don't use a hysteroscope, making the whole thing less complicated. But some experts warn against doing anything inside the uterus 'blind' – they believe the surgeon needs to see what's happening. There's a small risk of perforating the uterus, which research has shown is reduced when a hysteroscope is used.

First-generation methods require more specialized skill and therefore are offered by fewer surgeons. They are suitable for more complicated cases, for example where there are polyps, fibroids or sticky patches of scar-like tissue called adhesions. They may require a longer recovery time than later methods.

Second-generation methods are the ones usually recommended by NICE. They are simpler and therefore can be carried out by more surgeons who don't specialize. They are suitable for straightforward cases in which there is no abnormality other than the condition being treated. The presence of fibroids makes some techniques more difficult.

These operations are usually very brief and may allow you to go home the same day. Recovery is generally quick and problem-free, although you may have vaginal discharge for some days.

Ablation techniques are rapidly evolving, so ask your doctor about the different kinds available. Points to keep in mind are that glitches in the earlier methods may have been dealt with in the latest versions, and the techniques and equipment are being constantly refined. On the other hand, the older techniques have been more widely tested, their long-term effects are better known and surgeons have had more experience in carrying them out.

First-generation procedures

First-generation procedures to remove the endometrium are as follows:

- *Transcervical resection of the endometrium (TCRE).* This is the original method of removing the endometrium, through a hysteroscope with a wire loop at the end. A high-frequency electric current is passed through it to destroy the womb lining.
- *Rollerball ablation.* An electric current is conducted through a rollerball at the tip of the hysteroscope. Although this has some advantages, it does not allow polyps or fibroids to be removed unless a less common variant called a rollerbar, or barrel, is used.
- *Laser ablation.* The endometrium is vaporized by a tightly focused laser beam. Another version using a slightly different tool destroys the endometrium by coagulating it.
- *TCRE with Mirena.* Some research has shown that inserting an intrauterine system during a resection procedure is extra-effective in reducing heavy bleeding. This is not yet offered as a standard procedure.

Second-generation procedures

The number of second-generation ablation techniques is increasing all the time. Those shown here are the ones recommended by NICE in its 2007 guidelines, the latest available.

- *Thermal balloon ablation.* A balloon containing a heating element is inserted into the uterus and filled with fluid. The heat destroys the lining of the womb without harming anything around it.
- *Impedance-controlled bipolar radiofrequency ablation.* A sheath containing a bipolar radiofrequency electrode is placed in the uterus. The sheath is then pulled back, allowing the electrode to expand and fit the shape of the uterine cavity. The endometrium is then destroyed with radiofrequency energy before the electrode is retracted into the sheath and removed from the uterus.
- *Microwave endometrial ablation (MEA).* A microwave probe is inserted into the uterus and moved from side to side in order to destroy the lining.
- *Free-fluid thermal endometrial ablation.* The endometrium is destroyed by heated saline solution.

Laser surgery

This isn't the name of an operation, but a description of the equipment used in a range of operations for various conditions. Lasers are among the many different tools that can be used to remove the womb lining in endometrial ablation, for example, or to destroy a fibroid.

But it's often used to describe the clearance of womb-lining tissue that has grown outside the womb, in women who have endometriosis. It can also be used to remove adhesions: sticky patches of tissue resulting from endometriosis or from scarring, which can 'glue' abdominal organs together and cause intense pain.

Myolysis, or myoma coagulation

The aim of this procedure is to cut off the blood supply to a fibroid using heat or lasers, in order to shrink the fibroid. It can also be done by freezing the fibroid with liquid nitrogen, a procedure called cryomyolysis. It can be carried out through the vagina, so there is no incision or scar, or can be done laparoscopically, through a small incision in the abdomen.

These operations were pioneered in the late 1980s but are not widely used as they don't have a high success rate. They are only suitable for a few small fibroids. Although they aim to preserve fertility, they frequently leave internal scarring and adhesions that could lead to pregnancy complications.

Myomectomy

This is an operation to remove fibroids, leaving the uterus intact. If you have several large fibroids you will probably be offered an abdominal procedure, which requires a general anaesthetic. Approaching the uterus this way allows the surgeon space to find and remove all the fibroids.

Myomectomy can also be done through a smaller 'keyhole' incision in the abdomen, using a laparoscope and destroying the fibroids with either laser or electric current. But NICE guidelines show that this route is less effective and more risky; also, it is harder to remove large fibroids, which are the ones most likely to be causing symptoms. There's a small risk of the uterus being perforated or the operation leaving adhesions.

Small fibroids can be removed in a minimally invasive operation through the vagina, with the use of a hysteroscope.

Presacral neurectomy (PSN)

When no cause for pain can be discovered and treated, and the pain is severe, surgeons have the option of cutting a group of nerves in the lower back that carry pain signals from the uterus. Presacral neurectomy is also sometimes done during surgery for endometriosis. However, it can cause bladder and bowel problems. It is no longer widely used in the UK, as NICE guidelines state that it is not effective.

Radical trachelectomy

In some cases of cervical cancer that are caught early on, an operation called radical trachelectomy can be carried out as a less invasive procedure than a hysterectomy. This removes the cervix, leaving the rest of the womb and the ovaries intact. It may still be possible to become pregnant afterwards, and have the baby by Caesarean section.

Sacrohysteropexy

This is a procedure to treat uterine prolapse. The uterus is attached to the anterior longitudinal ligament over the sacrum and held in place with mesh. This can be done with a laparoscope or as open abdominal surgery.

Sacrospinous fixation

This is another operation to treat uterine prolapse, by attaching the uterus to the sacrospinous ligament on one side or both sides. Carried out via the vagina, it is less invasive than sacrohysteropexy, but it risks damaging nerves that can cause long-term pain in the buttocks and down the leg.

Ultrasound surgery

Guided by an MRI scanner, high-intensity sound waves are directed onto fibroids to destroy the tissue. This is a new treatment that hasn't yet been widely tested and therefore is not widely available.

Uterine artery embolization (UAE)

Originally devised to stop excessive bleeding after childbirth, this is now also used to reduce the size of fibroids and ease menorrhagia. The arteries feeding the fibroids are blocked with a grainy substance so that, deprived of their blood supply, the fibroids shrink. In the most successful cases they vanish altogether during the next few months, and in many cases they shrink to about half size.

However, it doesn't work for everyone. There is a small risk that it could cause premature menopause, and an even smaller risk of haemorrhage, infection or damage to the surrounding tissue. A 2006 Cochrane Collaboration report found that women tended to have more minor complications, such as vaginal discharge and nausea, after UAE than after hysterectomy. On the other hand they recovered and returned to work earlier after a UAE.

Uterine nerve ablation/uterosacral ligament resection

These two operations aim to relieve severe, long-standing pain that has not been relieved by medication. They involve cutting or burning the nerves in a small section of ligament attached to the uterus. NICE has stated that, like presacral neurectomy, they have not been found effective in the long term, so they are no longer frequently carried out in the UK.

8

Complementary and alternative medicine

Some of the oldest therapies in use today are complementary and alternative medicine (CAM). Until recently they were backed by nothing except long-standing tradition. Since about 1990, there's been a growing body of research into the effectiveness and safety of various CAM therapies. This has, of course, found that some are neither safe nor effective.

Studies funded by the manufacturers are more likely to find a product is worth using than studies by independent researchers. But exactly the same is true of drug trials. So the best evidence to look for is that carried out by charities, or by independent bodies such as the UK Medical Research Council or the US National Institutes of Health, or by university researchers who are not funded by manufacturers.

This chapter looks at remedies that have been found safe and effective in scientific studies, plus some gentle herbal helpers that are backed by long and harmless use.

Pain relief

Chronic pain is the most common symptom among the gynaecological conditions covered in this book. It takes many different forms: nagging pelvic discomfort, backache, sharp pangs, grinding pain, a dragging sensation, even the headaches caused by premenstrual syndrome. Other than cancer, these conditions are not life-threatening (except in unusual circumstances such as an unstoppable haemorrhage or a long-standing untreated infection, which require emergency care).

As long as your doctor has confirmed that the pain has a known cause, you have several options. You may seek treatment for the underlying condition, or keep it under control with self-help techniques, or leave it alone if your doctor agrees. Whichever path you take, there's no point putting up with pain when you don't have to.

Acupuncture has been found effective in easing pain, and may do so after as little as one session. The effects tend to wear off quite soon, but a series of treatments may give longer-lasting relief. It is believed to work by increasing the body's output of pain-relieving hormones, though medical science isn't clear about the exact mechanism. Practitioners insert needles into your skin, so you need to be very certain that they have a recognized qualification and meet strict standards of hygiene in order to avoid infection.

Acupressure has some of the same effects as acupuncture, but uses finger pressure instead of inserting needles. As a non-invasive treatment, it doesn't carry the health risks posed by insertion of needles.

Massage has a profound effect on backache and muscle pain – which itself is often caused by tension building up around pelvic pain. Tension is frequently held in the shoulders and down the back on each side of the spine. Although an in-depth massage can feel strenuous at the time, you should not have any pain afterwards other than, at most, some slight muscle soreness. The main effect, which should be noticeable after the first treatment, is pain relief and increased flexibility in muscles that you may not have realized were stiff with tension.

A *castor-oil compress* can relieve pain in the pelvis and breast and may also reduce inflammation. Take a thick, soft, clean cloth large enough to fold into several layers covering the painful area. A well-washed old plain T-shirt will also do, folded into eight layers. Pour castor oil on it and squeeze out any surplus so that it doesn't drip – castor oil leaves stains that won't wash out. Place the compress over your breast or abdomen, or lie on your front and put it on your lower back. Cover it with a piece of clean plastic, such as a carrier bag, and put a hot-water bottle or heating pad on top. Relax for up to an hour to let the warm oil do its soothing work. You can store the cloth and oil in a container in the fridge and reuse them.

Always get a diagnosis from your doctor if you are suffering from pain. Don't take for granted that it's either harmless or caused by a condition you already know about.

Herbal options

There are many herbal remedies on the market for gynaecological symptoms, but for most of them there is little evidence that they work. Some do seem to have strong effects, though, especially black cohosh, red clover and ginseng.

However, the strength of these herbs lies in their oestrogenic properties, which means that it's not safe to recommend them to anyone with oestrogen-fuelled diseases. Some people are convinced that they have beneficial effects, replacing harmful forms of oestrogen with a milder substitute. That hasn't yet been proved one way or the other. So it's not known for certain whether these herbs promote oestrogen-dependent cancers such as those of the breast, ovary or uterus – but it isn't worth taking the risk.

However, some other herbs have been found to help some of the symptoms you may encounter without disturbing oestrogen production.

- Evening primrose oil reduces breast pain and tenderness, along with some symptoms of PMS.
- Cranberry juice, as a drink or in capsules, has been found to prevent recurrent bladder infections such as cystitis.
- St John's wort can relieve the kind of mild depression caused by hormonal fluctuations. Be careful with it, as this powerful herb interacts with several drugs (especially antidepressants) and can make your skin oversensitive to the sun.
- Hops help you sleep: not when you drink them in the form of beer, but when you breathe their fragrance. Sew the dried flowers into a folded handkerchief to make a miniature pillow, and it should help you drift off to sleep.

Fresh from your garden

There's something very satisfying about plucking herbal helpers from your own garden or windowsill herb collection, or at least making them up from your kitchen cupboard. Several of these time-honoured remedies are used to tackle the symptoms of gynaecological conditions.

There's no overwhelming scientific evidence for most of these except lavender and peppermint. But small-scale trials have proved the benefits of most. And they are all traditional remedies that have stood the test of time.

- Lavender can help with a headache. Rub in your hands and inhale the smell, as this has been proved to reduce the pain.
- Rosemary increases blood flow to your brain, so it may help to clear the 'brain fog' caused by hormonal upheaval.
- Sage has been found to do its bit for the brain too, by improving memory in a series of tests.

A gentle way to take herbal remedies is as a tea, also known as a tisane or infusion. To make a tea, take a heaped teaspoonful or more of the herb. Most of those below are also widely available as tea bags, sometimes organic. Cover with boiling water, allow to cool to drinking temperature and then strain off to drink. If you wish, you can then cover the herb with more boiling water and make a second infusion too. If you are using a pot, make sure it's a new one that hasn't had ordinary tea brewed in it, so the boiling water doesn't pick up any tannin from inside the pot.

- Peppermint makes a gently soothing aid to digestion. It can relieve wind and other forms of indigestion except, possibly, heartburn, an acid feeling in mid-chest. (It's not recommended for heartburn, in which acid leaks upwards from the stomach into the oesophagus, because it is thought to weaken the valve that's meant to stop that happening.) Rubbed in your hands, the leaves release a smell that can relieve headaches.
- Camomile flowers are used to make a classic tea for stress, headaches and insomnia. Perfect for a bedtime drink, camomile tea may even counteract cramps. Add some ginger and cinnamon for a drink to relieve dysmenorrhoea.
- Lemon balm (melissa) has a pleasant fragrance, and is said to soothe anxiety and lift spirits.
- Cherry stalks, dried and used in an infusion, are mildly diuretic and are traditionally used to relieve cystitis. If you have a cherry tree in your garden, you can be sure the fruit hasn't been touched by pesticides; otherwise, buy organic.

Taking the tablets

Many different supplements have been claimed to relieve various gynaecological symptoms. But the studies are usually carried out with larger amounts than we're advised to take.

It's very easy to cause a vitamin imbalance by taking supplements, and some, such as vitamins A and E, have harmful long-term effects when taken in excessive amounts. The B vitamins are especially helpful for women: B1 has been proved to ease dysmenorrhoea and B6 combats PMS. But they should not be taken in isolation from each other: if you're taking B1 or B6, you should also have a complete B-complex supplement.

It's even easier to upset your body's mineral balance. Calcium has been found to relieve the psychological components of PMS, and magnesium eases many menstrual symptoms. But taking any mineral alone runs the risk of causing other symptoms – or worse, creating a mineral imbalance that can do harm without your realizing.

So the best advice is not to take vitamin supplements without a multivitamin, and especially don't take mineral supplements without a multivitamin and multimineral supplement. Never take more than the stated dose, and stop at once if you have side effects. Don't continue for more than three months if they're not helping substantially. Safest of all is to get plenty of these nutrients from fresh ingredients.

Safe supplements

Ask your doctor's advice before taking any complementary remedy or supplement, and make sure your doctor knows what you're taking. Remember that herbs and supplements can clash with both prescription and over-the-counter drugs. Check this with your doctor and also at recognized medical sites online for added certainty, as your doctor can't be expected to know everything about non-orthodox therapies. If either of them recommends caution, don't take the product.

CAM for cancer

Complementary remedies – those that aim to work alongside orthodox medicine – have much to offer people with cancer. Therapies such as herbs and acupuncture have a remarkable list of healing qualities for pain, nausea and many other symptoms.

Studies have shown that meditation, relaxation and music therapy can relieve cancer patients' unhappiness and anxiety. Massage can provide an effective source of pain relief, as can acupuncture and hypnotherapy. Both acupuncture and hypnotherapy can also reduce the nausea caused by chemotherapy – wrist bands specially made to target acupressure points can be worn in hospital.

However, these work at reducing the symptoms. They're in a different category from alternative remedies: those that are claimed to work *instead of* conventional treatment.

'Help' that harms

Please don't waste time trying alternative remedies if you have had a cancer diagnosis. No shaman, herbalist, homoeopath or other alternative practitioner has ever been proved to cure a cancer. No 'psychic surgeon' has ever shown evidence of removing a real cancer from anyone's body, though you have to admire their skill with conjuring tricks.

Don't believe anyone claiming that their products can either heal cancer or stop it growing. Although various plant foods may reduce your risk of developing cancer, no product made from them has been proved effective: you have to eat the foods as part of a healthy diet.

Natural remedies can work wonders for long-term health and everyday ailments. Along with exercise and healthy eating, they may even reduce your risk of major diseases, including cancer. But once a cancer has developed, it's in a different league. And any time you spend trying out such remedies is time the cancer is growing and spreading.

CAM research on the internet

The internet is both the world's greatest research tool and a breeding ground for myths and hoaxes. It is almost impossible to police, so anyone can claim or sell pretty much anything, backed with completely fictitious evidence. It takes very simple skills to create a professional-looking website, so that's no indication whether the content is true, semi-accurate or total fantasy.

You can buy all kinds of drugs and other remedies on the internet that are not legally sold in, for example, the European Union, because they have not been proved safe or effective. There's no quality control of any kind, so buying remedies on the internet isn't recommended, especially from sites based outside your own country. You have no way of checking whether they're genuine or even safe.

Many websites exist to promote someone's products or services. These may be valuable, or dangerous, or something in between – but without doing a lot of research, it's hard to find out. Others belong to individuals or organizations that promote unproven alternative ideas – often with the best intentions but little genuine knowledge. On the other hand, many blogs on CAM subjects have postings from people reporting their own experiences. And some of the patient-group websites have forums in which people discuss both orthodox and CAM treatments they've used. As well as reading what other people have found out, you can ask questions of your own and usefully share experiences.

CAM is harder to check than orthodox medicine, as less research has been carried out on it, although researchers are now starting to respond to the growing interest in alternatives. Some of the better-known subjects such as acupuncture may be covered on the mainstream charities' websites. You can also use the search methods detailed in Chapter 5, such as finding out if the Cochrane Collaboration or other major body has reported on the condition or technique you're interested in. And there are some independent CAM research sites, such as the following:

- NHS Complementary and Alternative Medicine Specialist Library <www.library.nhs.uk/CAM/>
- US National Center for Complementary and Alternative Medicine <http://nccam.nih.gov/>
- Australian Centre for Complementary Medicine Education and Research <www.uq.edu.au/accmer/>

9

For and against hysterectomy

When you have a long-standing health complaint that's been bringing you down for years, it's tempting to take any way out that's offered. Some women, by the time they reach the stage of seeking treatment, just want to be rid of the organ that's causing the trouble. That's one very good reason to seek help and advice early on, when you still have time and energy to look at alternatives. Another good reason, of course, is that far more can be done when conditions are diagnosed in good time. Most hysterectomies are carried out for conditions that are not life-threatening.

Even so, some women don't like the idea of taking long-term medication. Or they may suspect that newer techniques are not so well tested as hysterectomies. And in countries such as the United States, where about one-third of all women have lost their uterus by the time they reach 60, it may just seem like the natural thing to do. However, it's worth remembering that a hysterectomy does more than simply remove the source of your pain and debility. Having an internal organ removed can cause problems of its own. Apart from anything else, it changes your internal structure, and could lead to other organs prolapsing.

Ovaries and the loss of oestrogen

It's also important to consider whether your ovaries can be saved. The long-term side effects of hysterectomy are more severe if the ovaries are removed along with the uterus.

Most of the oestrogen in your body is produced by the ovaries. If you are still menstruating, having your ovaries removed will cause immediate menopause. Although oestrogen may be causing your present health problems, its sudden disappearance causes huge hormonal upheaval. It's very different from the natural process of perimenopause, which happens over a period of years, giving your body time to adjust.

Weighing up the options

Apart from the relief you hope for, operations can cause side effects in both the short term and the long term. Hysterectomy tends to have larger effects – for both good and bad – as it's a more serious operation than the alternatives. However, the other options also have effects you need to consider.

Do all the research you can before making a decision. That could include reading this book, questioning your doctor, talking to other women who have faced similar decisions, contacting patients' groups and searching for answers online. Below are some of the factors to take into account.

Possible immediate side effects

Hysterectomy is major surgery, and takes longer to recover from than most of the smaller alternatives. About one woman in ten will need further treatment, most commonly antibiotics for an infection. See Chapter 11 for more details on recovery.

During the operation itself, there is a small risk of thrombosis, infection, haemorrhage needing a blood transfusion, or a return to theatre for more stitches. Any operation can go wrong, but there is only a very small risk of death: less than one in 1,000. Also during the operation there is a risk of damage to the bladder, ureters or bowel. Perhaps surprisingly, bladder damage is more likely to happen with a laparoscopic hysterectomy than with the traditional method.

The risk continues after the operation, because the uterus is joined to the bladder and rectum by bands of stretchy tissue called ligaments, so its removal can damage these other organs. In the worst cases, this can cause incontinence of the bladder or bowel.

If you had the operation to remove a prolapsed uterus, it's not uncommon for the top of your vagina to sag afterwards: a condition known as vaginal vault prolapse. This happens in about 15 per cent of cases. It's a rare side effect if you had the hysterectomy for other reasons. But other neighbouring organs may also prolapse without the uterus in place.

Other options

Any of the surgical alternatives to hysterectomy also carry a small risk of harm and require time to heal. The risks and healing time are less than for hysterectomy, as the other operations are smaller. Any operation that's carried out vaginally may cause some damage to the vagina.

The end of fertility

After a hysterectomy, your periods will stop and you will no longer be able to become pregnant. The eggs your ovaries produce each month will simply be reabsorbed into the body. There's a theoretical possibility that one could be fertilized, but as there is nowhere for the fertilized egg to be implanted or nourished, it would again simply be reabsorbed.

If you have kept your ovaries, a surrogate mother could, in theory, have one of your eggs implanted and carry the baby for you. Remember, though, that hysterectomy often damages the ovaries, which may no longer work effectively afterwards. If your ovaries are being removed because of cancer, you could have your eggs frozen and stored beforehand, with the possibility of finding a surrogate mother in the future. However, the chance of a successful pregnancy in either case is not very high. It's realistic to consider that you will not be able to have children after a hysterectomy.

Other options

Many of the alternative operations in this book, especially those for fibroids, will also put an end to any chance of childbearing. You cannot have children after any form of endometrial ablation or resection, as this is meant to destroy the lining of the uterus. Many women stop having periods altogether after this treatment (although this doesn't mean they're going through the menopause, as their ovaries are still producing oestrogen). In the rare event that an egg is fertilized, it cannot be brought to term and you risk a life-threatening ectopic pregnancy.

Myomectomy, myolysis and uterine artery embolization (UAE) aim to preserve fertility by destroying fibroids without harming the womb. But in reality, they are likely to reduce your chance of a successful pregnancy. Unless you are certain that fibroids are stopping you conceiving or carrying a pregnancy to term, you have a better chance of giving birth if you don't have them operated on.

If you still hope to have children, it's important to let your doctor know, and discuss the consequences of any treatment.

The process of grief

Mourning is a side effect that takes many women by surprise. Although it may have caused years of illness, the womb plays a central part in many women's view of themselves, and they feel less feminine without it. Whether or not you have had children, or wanted to have more, you may be startled by a feeling of loss. Of course, you are no less a woman than when your uterus was in place, but emotions don't always listen to sense.

This side effect is much more likely if your ovaries have also been removed. Loss of ovaries has a far larger effect physically, and therefore is more likely to cause psychological problems in adjustment. Even a natural menopause arouses some feelings of sadness and loss in most women, even if briefly. When menopause is triggered abruptly, and earlier in life than expected, such feelings are bound to be more extreme.

The mourning process is helped enormously if the operation has solved your long-standing health problems. And many women feel as unburdened by hysterectomy as they would from having a painful tooth out. On the other hand, you may feel cheated if the operation didn't help as much as you'd expected. So make sure you know in advance how much improvement you should expect, both as soon as you've recovered from surgery and in the longer term.

Other options

You may also feel a sense of loss after having alternative operations that end or reduce your fertility. Many other operations have a lower success rate than hysterectomy, so you are more likely to feel 'cheated'.

New symptoms

Many women report new symptoms after a hysterectomy. New pain is common (see below). Other than that, the symptoms are often emotional or psychological, such as depression, mood swings and anxiety.

In some cases, the symptoms are related to feelings of uncertainty or regret about the operation. The best way of preventing this is to do all possible research beforehand, get second or third opinions where necessary, make yourself as well informed as possible, and only go ahead with the operation if you are certain that it is the best decision in your circumstances. In other cases, symptoms are caused by hormonal upheaval. If they don't settle down within a few months, you may need to see your doctor again.

Other women report headaches, heart palpitations, exhaustion, urinary infections and other physical symptoms. These could also be hormone-related, possibly because the hysterectomy has triggered the perimenopause – the changes leading up to the menopause. If you are perimenopausal, hormone replacement therapy (HRT) may help.

Symptoms could also arise from damage to other organs caused by the hysterectomy. A small number of women report that they develop arthritis soon after the hysterectomy, possibly because damage to the ovaries may have reduced their supply of hormones that protect the joints.

In all cases, you should see your doctor about any new symptoms.

Other options

Other procedures are less likely to trigger the perimenopause, as they should not damage blood supply to the ovaries. However, it can still happen. Laparoscopic operations (whether hysterectomy or others) have a slightly higher chance of damaging the surrounding organs.

Pain

Although no operation can be guaranteed to be 100 per cent safe and successful, hysterectomy seems to leave many women disappointed.

Long-standing pelvic pain is one of the major reasons for having a hysterectomy. However, the operation isn't guaranteed to cure pain, especially if doctors had not been able to find out exactly what was causing it. And in recent years it has been discovered that many women develop chronic pain after a hysterectomy when they hadn't suffered much pain before. Researchers contacting women a year or more after hysterectomy have been surprised to discover a quarter to a third of them suffering chronic pain. In a recent study, one woman in eight suffered pain more than two days a week, and pain started after the hysterectomy for one in seven.

You're most at risk of having chronic pain after a hysterectomy if your main problem before the operation was pelvic pain, with no clear diagnosis. Your risk is also raised if you've given birth to more than two children or had a Caesarean, and if you suffer from pain in other parts of your body. The risk seems to be lower if you have spinal rather than general anaesthesia.

Other options

You may suffer pain after other operations described in this book. As they are less likely to give a complete cure, you may also have to go through them more than once.

Your sex life

This may be changed for better or worse by a hysterectomy. If your symptoms made sex painful or difficult before, a successful hysterectomy could solve the problem. That's why many women report that having the operation was as good for their sex lives as for their health. However, the removal of your uterus can have further effects, and you need to be aware of the risks in advance.

During the first few weeks of recovery, you should avoid sexual intercourse as you are still healing inside. After that, some women are worried by the fact that they can't see how their internal wounds are healing – it may not feel safe. Do check with your doctor how long you should refrain from intercourse: it's not the same for everyone, and will depend on how well you're healing.

In the longer term, be prepared for a hysterectomy to cause some changes in your sexual responsiveness. The very complex network of nerves and fine blood vessels in the pelvic area can easily be damaged. The effect on your glands could reduce your natural lubrication, and any damage to your vagina could make it less able to expand and contract. The risk of damage is greater if your cervix was removed along with your uterus.

Your ovaries are the main source of the hormones governing arousal and sexual pleasure. Even if your ovaries are not removed, they may no longer be functioning at full power, as the operation can easily damage them or reduce their blood supply. Many women report a lower libido after a hysterectomy, even if they kept their ovaries. There are remedies, including hormone replacement therapy (HRT), but you should be prepared for this sudden change.

Women who could feel the uterus contracting during orgasm will no longer have that pleasure after hysterectomy. Some women enjoy the feeling of their partner's penis bumping their cervix during intercourse, although others find it uncomfortable. Either way, this will be gone after hysterectomy, unless your cervix is still in place.

If your ovaries have also been removed, you will be menopausal and your remaining internal sex organs will be bereft of oestrogen. Your vagina will become shorter, and you'll stop producing the natural lubrication that makes sex comfortable and enjoyable. You'll be advised to take HRT – just the oestrogen component, as hysterectomy removes the need for progestogen to protect the uterus.

Other options

Any vaginal procedure runs a small risk of damaging the vagina. Other operations are less likely than hysterectomy to reduce the functioning of the ovaries, though it is still possible.

Long-term effects

Your menopause is likely to happen earlier, on average, than if you did not have a hysterectomy. You are more likely to develop osteoporosis – brittle bones – after a hysterectomy, and so be at risk of fractures. The likelihood is greatly increased if your ovaries have been removed. But you are less likely to suffer from certain cancers.

The other long-term results of hysterectomy are less definite. Some studies have shown that women who have had a hysterectomy go on to live an average-length life. But others point to the increased risk of heart disease, which becomes much more common after menopause: your heart starts deteriorating sooner if a hysterectomy has caused early menopause.

If your ovaries have also been removed, the effects are clearer. You have a greater risk of dementia and your life expectancy is slightly shorter than if you had not had the operation.

Other options

Little is known about the long-term effects of new operations. Any surgery in the area runs the risk of damaging the ovaries, or their nerves or blood supply, so there is a possibility of premature menopause. However, these operations are not expected to have such marked effects as hysterectomy or oophorectomy (removal of ovaries). Their main disadvantage, compared with removal of the womb or ovaries, is that they are less likely to provide a complete cure.

Questions to ask about hysterectomy

Ask your doctor

- Are you certain what is causing my symptoms?
- Is my condition likely to be relieved by the menopause, if it's not treated?
- Have you carried out tests (for example a hysteroscopy) that clearly show what is inside my uterus?
- What are the chances of complete success? Or how much will it help?

- What are the risks?
- How is this likely to affect my sex life?

Ask yourself

- How much is this condition bothering me?
- Is there anything about a hysterectomy that's likely to be worse than living with my condition?
- Do I want to have (more) children?
- Have I given the alternatives a chance?

The chances of success

Hysterectomy should cure adenomyosis, dysmenorrhoea, endometrial hyperplasia, fibroids in the womb, heavy bleeding and polyps. Other operations for these conditions have a lower chance of success, and may have to be repeated. Some women have alternative operations more than once, and end up having a hysterectomy anyway. Although hysterectomy obviously cures uterine prolapse, it may cause (or reveal) other prolapses. A hysterectomy may need to be carried out if PID or endometriosis has caused too much damage to save the uterus. But as both these conditions affect organs outside the uterus, you may still have trouble with them afterwards.

About one woman in ten will find that a hysterectomy does not solve her problem. This is most likely if she has endometriosis, or if her main problem was chronic pelvic pain that could not be traced to any specific cause. Also, it may not put an end to premenstrual syndrome unless your ovaries are also removed, as PMS is caused by sensitivity to hormones that the ovaries will still be producing. If you are sensitive to hormonal fluctuations, the changes caused by surgical menopause after your ovaries are removed may produce similar symptoms, although these should be temporary. If any of this applies to you, it is especially wise to try all the options first, particularly the self-help measures.

Shout about pain

If you have chronic pain, push for all available tests to get a diagnosis. It could be caused by something unrelated to your reproductive system, which might be curable.

Don't agree to a hysterectomy just to see if it will work. Undiagnosed pain is the condition for which hysterectomy is most likely to be unsuccessful. You may lose your uterus for no good reason, while missing the chance to cure your real condition.

Removal of the ovaries, later, sometimes brings relief for endometriosis and for PMS when hysterectomy alone has not done enough.

When hysterectomy is the only answer

The factors to weigh up for or against hysterectomy are only relevant if you are dealing with a condition that is not going to kill you. If you have cancer and your doctor recommends a hysterectomy, please don't waste time. It's always worth getting a second opinion, from an equally qualified specialist, if you're not sure about the first doctor's advice. But if hysterectomy is going to save your life, there's no other choice worth taking.

This doesn't mean that you have to abandon all gentle natural or self-help therapies. On the contrary, these are very valuable, both to build you up before the operation and to optimize your healthy future afterwards. Read Chapter 8 on CAM to find out more.

Occasionally, other conditions make a hysterectomy unavoidable. Sometimes there's no other way of stopping a haemorrhage before you would bleed to death. And rare cases of long-standing PID may prove resistant even to injections of powerful antibiotics.

Those are life-threatening circumstances. But even if your life isn't in danger, a hysterectomy may turn out to be the best answer in the end.

Making your choice

For conditions that aren't going to kill you, it's a question of doing the research, getting a range of advice, and making a well-informed decision. You can work through the self-help measures, the medicines, the minor operations. You'll almost certainly get some relief. But if it's not enough, and if all else has failed, only you can decide whether you would rather live with the symptoms or choose a hysterectomy.

Making a well-informed choice is an empowering decision. Having a hysterectomy under those circumstances is very different from being rushed into it for inadequate reasons and regretting it when you found out what you could have done instead.

Your uterus is an internal organ – no more, no less. Even if your ovaries also have to be removed, you haven't lost anything you can't live without. They are no more essential to your femininity, or your personality, than your appendix is. You have had a health problem, and solved it by the best means available. Now you have your life back, like anyone else after an operation or illness. No longer being weakened by ill health, you may find life far more complete and rewarding than before.

10

Hysterectomy options

The large majority of hysterectomies are carried out as 'elective' operations: you have chosen to have your uterus removed, rather than being forced into it by a life-threatening disease or emergency. As long as it's a freely made and well-informed choice, this is a positive move. Only you can decide how long you can put up with endless heavy bleeding or pain undermining your health and vitality. If the relief brought by natural menopause is far in the future, you may not wish to sacrifice another decade or more.

Hysterectomy is a very common operation. About a fifth of all British women and a third of American women have had their uterus removed by the time they reach 60. Although it is now considered that far too many hysterectomies are carried out, this does have an advantage if you need to have one. It means that the surgeon who operates on you is likely to be very experienced.

As with any operation, you have to weigh up several factors. New techniques have the advantage of being fine-tuned by surgeons who have learned from the shortcomings of traditional procedures. But they don't yet have years of evidence to show whether their results are better or worse. A surgeon who prefers older methods may be a stick-in-the-mud, or just cautious with other people's internal organs.

Evidence about new techniques is changing all the time. Ask your specialist for the latest statistics and information. (If they're not willing to help your research, why not?) Only you can assess the specialists and options available in your individual circumstances. If it isn't urgent, take some time to ask questions.

- Do the benefits of a new technique outweigh the lack of evidence for its long-term safety and effectiveness?
- Does a surgeon's long experience in carrying out a traditional operation outweigh any now known disadvantages?
- Is a surgeon who's keen to try out new methods likely to be a bit less cautious about risks?

Different routes: abdominal, laparoscopic or vaginal?

As in other areas of gynaecology, new techniques and knowledge have provided a range of options when a hysterectomy is needed. In many cases, surgeons can remove the womb through the vagina. They can also use 'keyhole' surgery, which doesn't leave a noticeable abdominal scar.

Laparotomy, or open abdominal surgery, is the traditional method. Cutting open the abdomen provides the most space for manoeuvre and the clearest view, both inside and outside the uterus, without special instruments. The downside is that it's major surgery, which leaves a large scar and needs a long recovery time.

However, laparotomy is still the most suitable for some purposes. If the uterus is very bulky, for example because it contains large fibroids, this is the only way of removing it. And if the operation is to remove cancer or endometriosis, this offers the best chance of getting it all out safely. It's also easier to remove the ovaries and fallopian tubes through the abdomen.

Many surgeons still do abdominal hysterectomies when they have a choice. Like anyone else, surgeons prefer to do what they're used to and what they're good at. If you'd rather have vaginal surgery and your specialist isn't keen, ask for a second opinion to find out whether another method would be suitable for you. You may need to have this operation carried out by someone else.

Laparoscopic or 'keyhole' surgery uses instruments and cameras on slender tubes passed through tiny incisions in the abdomen. It still allows the surgeon to see outside as well as inside the uterus. It has become popular for many operations since the technology became widely available in the 1990s, as it is much less invasive and leaves barely visible scars. However, keyhole surgery is not necessarily the best for a hysterectomy. The procedure takes longer than either abdominal or vaginal surgery and is more likely to damage the bladder or ureters. It should only be carried out by someone who specializes in surgery by this route.

Vaginal surgery is now recommended in most cases when the womb is a normal size and there's no cancer or endometriosis. It leaves no scar and should lead to a quick recovery. However, some women have reported damage to their vagina after this operation, making sexual activity painful. Ask your specialist about the risk of this in your case.

A laparoscopically assisted vaginal hysterectomy aims to give the best of both worlds. The keyhole instruments allow the surgeon to see the area surrounding the uterus without cutting open the abdomen.

The uterus is then removed through the vagina. But again, research has found more complications after laparoscopic procedures have been used.

Safety first

Preparing for your operation reduces the risk of adverse effects. Ask your doctor for a checklist of things to do before the operation.

- If you're taking certain medicines, you may need to stop them before the operation. But don't stop any medication unless your doctor says to do so.
- If you are very overweight, losing weight before the operation will reduce your risk of adverse effects. Don't go on a crash diet, as this does more harm than good. Ask your specialist if you have time to lose weight and if it's advisable.
- Giving up smoking will also reduce your risks, during any operation.

Extent of surgery

A hysterectomy may involve removing less than the entire uterus, or considerably more. How much depends on the reason for the operation. If it's for cancer, you need to get rid of everything that is or may be affected. But if it's to remove troublesome fibroids or put an end to heavy bleeding, for example, you have many more options.

Subtotal (partial or supracervical) hysterectomy

The uterus is removed but the cervix is left in place. This is a simpler operation, with little risk of side effects, and it can be done even if the ovaries are removed. The uterus can't be removed through your vagina if the cervix remains in place, so this has to be done through the abdomen.

If you're not at high risk of cervical cancer, it's worth asking if this would be suitable for you. Not all research supports the belief that it causes less disturbance to the surrounding organs than a total hysterectomy. However, many women feel more comfortable with it and find that it has less effect on their enjoyment of sex.

Total hysterectomy

This is the most common procedure. The entire uterus is removed, along with the cervix.

Hysterectomy with salpingo-oophorectomy

One or both ovaries and fallopian tubes are removed, together with the uterus and cervix. Bilateral salpingo-oophorectomy means removal of both ovaries and both fallopian tubes; unilateral salpingo-oophorectomy is removal of just one ovary and its tube.

This should only be done if your ovaries need to be removed because of cancer or severe polycystic ovary syndrome (PCOS). NICE's recommendation is not to remove ovaries and fallopian tubes except for real medical reasons. It should not be done to prevent a possible future cancer in someone who is at only average risk.

Radical (or Wertheim's) hysterectomy

The removal of the uterus, cervix, part of the upper vagina and lymph glands, often along with the ovaries and fallopian tubes, this operation is only done for cancer.

What about my ovaries?

The only condition in which it's essential to remove an ovary (oophorectomy) is ovarian cancer. Even then, if only one ovary is affected you may be able to keep the other one. They are also sometimes removed if a condition such as PCOS proves impossible to control any other way.

Until recently, about half of all women in their forties or older having a hysterectomy had their ovaries removed at the same time. This was to prevent any risk of ovarian cancer, even if the woman was not in a high-risk group. Hysterectomy with removal of healthy ovaries is still quite common now.

However, oophorectomy causes immediate menopause, with all the problems and symptoms that entails. Women going through a normal menopause have the choice of whether to use hormone replacement therapy (HRT) or not, but when menopause is so sudden it's hard to cope without it. And replacing the loss of oestrogen from the ovaries with HRT causes problems of its own.

Recent research has shown that unless they're endangering your life losing your ovaries does more harm than good, at least in women who are under 65 at the time of the operation. The increased risk of death from heart disease heavily outweighs the reduced risk of death from ovarian cancer. There's also a steep increase in osteoporosis and the risk of broken bones.

Some recent research (2007) has shown that women whose ovaries are removed are more prone to dementia and to a neurodegenerative condition called parkinsonism, and likely to develop these at an earlier age than average. Women who had lost both ovaries before the age of 42, researchers found, were nearly twice as likely as average to develop dementia. It's one of the many effects caused by the loss of hormones produced by the ovaries. And the ovaries are now known to go on producing small amounts of helpful hormones for years, or decades, after a natural menopause.

It is now considered wise not to remove ovaries unnecessarily. So if your hysterectomy is for a condition that's not life-threatening, you don't have PCOS and you are not at high risk of ovarian cancer, you should check with your surgeon that an oophorectomy is not planned as well. If it is, ask what the reason is and get a second opinion.

11

Recovering from a pelvic operation

If a hysterectomy has saved your life – congratulations! This should be the beginning of a happier and healthier chapter of your life. The same is true if you weighed up your options and chose a hysterectomy or other operation to cure symptoms that you had endured for too long. Chapter 9 has given you an idea of the after-effects of hysterectomy and of other surgical options. This chapter looks at ways of speeding your recovery, physically, emotionally and sexually.

Physical recovery

You'll need time to recover from a hysterectomy, whichever option you choose. Plan for at least six weeks off work, after which time you should have had your first post-operative check-up. Don't return to work until your doctor says so, because skimping on recovery time can slow down the healing process. And 'work' doesn't just mean a paid job – you shouldn't be doing housework or anything strenuous for some weeks. Some women will need up to three months off work.

Open abdominal surgery has the most impact, and you may find it hard to walk for the first few weeks. Laparoscopic and vaginal surgery are kinder to your abdominal muscles, but in other respects the process is similar. You may be surprised by the amount of time it takes to regain any strength and energy.

Constipation and wind are problems for many women in the first few weeks after a hysterectomy. Eating fruit may increase the flatulence, but you still need plenty of fibre to counteract constipation, so eat as many fresh vegetables as possible. Straining to open your bowel is not only painful but dangerous when you've just had stitches, so drink as much as you can to keep your motions soft.

As codeine-based painkillers cause constipation, see if your doctor can recommend an alternative, such as ibuprofen. If natural remedies aren't working quickly enough, you may be offered laxatives. Even if you generally prefer to avoid medicaments, a small dose of a gentle laxative is better than risking the harm caused by constipation after a hysterectomy.

You should need less time to recover from other pelvic operations, as you will not have lost an internal organ. Your doctor will tell you how long you should rest. However, don't push yourself. You have still had an invasive procedure and the wounds inside need to heal.

Doctors no longer encourage people to lie down for long after an operation. The sooner you start to move again after any operation, the lower your risk of harmful effects such as thrombosis. Easy movement, such as walking, also helps your bowel start working again naturally.

You're likely to be given some gentle exercises to strengthen your pelvic floor and improve circulation in your abdomen. Do these as often as you're advised to, in order to speed up healing. As soon as you can comfortably move, check with your doctor how much you can safely walk during the day. Strolling through pleasant scenery is an excellent way of nurturing yourself while getting a little exercise.

Don't be tempted to go out in the car, even as a passenger, until your wounds have healed. Six weeks after a hysterectomy is a rule of thumb, but you will know it's too soon if you flinch at the very thought of a seatbelt! Whatever operation you've had, you shouldn't consider driving yourself until you would be able to do an emergency stop without pain.

A small percentage of women develop complications after any of the operations described in this book. You may even need to go back to hospital for further treatment. There's only a very small risk of this, but you do need to keep follow-up appointments so that your doctor can ensure everything is healing as it's meant to.

Stay alert for infections

It's normal to have some discharge for the first few weeks after a hysterectomy, and this may happen to a lesser extent after other operations too. Using pads rather than tampons reduces the risk of infection. But do stay alert for any danger signs. Let your doctor know if you experience any of the following:

- The discharge becomes heavy or develops an unpleasant smell.
- The discharge becomes bright red.
- Your wound feels hot or tender.
- The scar looks sore or red.
- You need to urinate frequently.
- You have pain when urinating.

Emotional recovery

You may feel a sense of loss after the operation – and not only if your womb or ovaries were removed. Some of the alternatives also put an end to your chance of having children, and loss of fertility can be equally hard to deal with. There's a big difference between not planning to become pregnant, and knowing that you can't become pregnant.

If you had a hysterectomy, with or without oophorectomy, you're also dealing with the loss of an internal organ. The psychological impact of losing a body part can be out of all proportion to what other people would see as its importance.

Grief may take you by surprise, especially if you were looking forward to getting the operation over with. Don't try to bully yourself out of it – much less let anyone else do so. Go easy on yourself as you come to terms with this loss. Having an anaesthetic can also make you feel quite strange and emotionally off-balance for a while afterwards, so give yourself time to recover.

Some women find it helpful to write a letter to the children they won't have. Some even write to their ovaries or womb, thanking them for the children they've created or sheltered, or apologizing for no longer wanting them. This may sound weird, but no one else has to know, and it's a simple way of getting it off your mind. Then burn the letter, or tear it up and bury it in the garden, and forget about it.

It's harder to move on if the operation has been less successful than you hoped. That's where it's helpful to have made a fully informed decision and chosen an appropriate option. Nothing is guaranteed in life. You haven't done something stupid and let yourself down, and you haven't been wronged. That makes it easier to accept the results. You'll continue your research, and when the time is right, you'll decide on your next step.

Meanwhile do read through the self-help chapters in this book and see if there's anything else you could be doing for yourself. You may find that even if your problem hasn't been totally solved your symptoms may have been reduced to the extent that self-help measures make them easy to live with.

If you find you are grieving for more than a few days, you'll need to work through it as you work through any other pain or loss in life. Talk it through with understanding friends, or seek counselling from a psychologist specializing in a short-term process such as cognitive behaviour therapy (CBT). Don't let the mourning process drag on and become an unhealthy, depressing habit.

Sexual recovery

One of the benefits of having an operation to solve pain or heavy bleeding is that it can restore your sex life. Few things are less conducive to sexual arousal than sharp or grinding pain, or the exhaustion caused by endless loss of blood. If you are single, you may even have given up on trying to have a sex life.

You don't have to wait till everything's healed inside to start enjoying foreplay and other kinds of intimacy again. Just don't have sexual intercourse until you're certain that it can't cause any internal damage. Six weeks after a hysterectomy is the usual embargo. For other operations, especially those carried out vaginally, wait until you can't feel any soreness.

What if the physical problem has cleared up, but you're just not interested any more? Surveys carried out on women's sexuality after hysterectomy have reported that the operation doesn't generally reduce women's libido or their ability to enjoy sex. But this doesn't tally with the experience of many women, who find that their sex drive has died off since they underwent hysterectomy.

That's to be expected when the ovaries are also removed. Ovaries are the main source not only of oestrogen but also of the 'male' hormone testosterone, which women also produce in smaller amounts and which fuels our sex drive. Hysterectomy without oophorectomy isn't meant to affect the ovaries. But in reality, the fact that women reach menopause sooner, on average, after a hysterectomy makes it pretty clear that in many cases the ovaries' ability to function has been reduced.

Although there's less risk of damage to the ovaries with alternative operations, it can still happen. Loss of sex drive could then also be a warning sign that perimenopause may be starting. Additionally, any procedure carried out via the vagina can damage the intricate network of nerves and blood vessels in the area. This could blunt sensation, weaken vaginal muscles or reduce lubrication. The vagina may be slower or less effective in expanding and lubricating to welcome the penis. This can make sex painful, which negates much of the benefit from the operation.

Luckily, all these problems have been widely studied and there's a plethora of solutions.

Reawakening your pleasure in sex

Testosterone is available on prescription, as are drugs that aim to increase blood circulation to the clitoris. These may not be an answer, as women's sexual response is more complex than men's and is affected by many other factors than just the physical. And any drugs carry the risk of unwanted side effects.

However, there are also products to stimulate the genital area, such as suction devices, vibrators and sex toys. Why not look in at one of the growing number of erotic suppliers that provide all kinds of novelties to liven up your sex life? You can find them on the average high street and they make a point of appealing to women with fun and fantasy. The online possibilities are endless too.

As women's sexual arousal is much less genitally centred than men's, you may find that products provide only part of the answer. For most women, sexual intercourse is just part of a whole experience that may involve stimulation of all or any part of the body, along with emotion, fantasy, playfulness and much else. You may be more aroused by massage, or games, or bathing with your partner.

If sex has been a long-standing problem because of your gynaecological condition, you may need time to rebuild your confidence, and possibly also your relationship with your partner. Give yourselves time to learn to relax and enjoy each other again. If pain has soured your pleasure in your body, it may take months for fear to be fully replaced by enjoyment.

Whatever happens, don't accept that your sex life is over, unless you want it to be. The operation you've had is meant to solve the problems that may have reduced your ability to enjoy sex. Even if you've had a radical hysterectomy and your ovaries have also been removed, it shouldn't be the end of your sexuality. Speak to your doctor, or ask to be referred to a specialist if the self-help options haven't done enough to improve matters.

Essential lubrication

If your problem is that the glands around your vagina no longer produce abundant lubrication, do sort this out as soon as you notice. Left untreated, vaginal dryness makes sex painful and unwelcome. Over a period of time, you or your partner will notice that you're less likely to initiate sex and more likely to find an excuse for not taking part. You may even start physically avoiding your partner, who is likely to feel hurt and rejected. If you don't want to talk about it, your relationship could go downhill sharply.

Luckily, this problem is very easy to solve, so please don't leave it a moment longer than necessary. Vaginal dryness is a normal result of natural menopause too, and manufacturers have seized the chance to supply a wide range of options to this ever-growing market. Lubricants are readily available from pharmacists and specialist shops now, in numerous formulations. Do take the time to find some that suit both you and your partner. You may find one brand more comfortable for use on your vulva, while your partner prefers the feel of another one inside – buy a basketful and experiment! There's even an organic version available (see 'Useful addresses').

Very few products have made a bigger difference to mature women's sex lives and relationships. Lubrication is as valuable as contraception, and has probably saved more than a few marriages.

Importantly, these products don't just rescue your sex life. Vaginal dryness is uncomfortable, often causing soreness and itchiness. It increases the incidence of thrush, cystitis and other painful infections. These in turn can become a recurrent nuisance that is harder to treat every time, and may go on to cause internal damage as serious as kidney failure.

Another range of products called vaginal moisturizers are for regular use, whether you are sexually active or not. Available over the counter, online and in some cases on prescription, they are applied two or three times a week to keep the vagina comfortable and healthy. Some are recommended for insertion in the morning; you may feel more confident wearing a pad the first time, just in case of any leakage. You can, of course, tailor the amount you use to your own needs and comfort.

You can choose from various delivery systems such as pessaries or gels, with or without an applicator. There's even one made from soya. As with lubricants, they're available in so many different formulations that it's worth trying several. Vaginal moisturizers can also be used as lubricants for love-making. You and your partner may find they're too slippery, or this may add to your enjoyment – try it and see!

Another good reason to reduce stress

Hormonal changes triggered by damage to the ovaries tend to be more abrupt than those that happen during the natural process of menopause. Part of the reason is that the perimenopause takes several years, during which time the ovaries slowly reduce their output of hormones. This gives other sources time to increase their output – not to the same level as a younger woman's ovaries, but enough to ease the transition.

The adrenal glands normally produce small amounts of both oestrogen and testosterone. But when you're under long-term pressure, these hormones lose out to constant production of the stress hormone cortisol. So learning to relax could give your body a chance to ease off the stress hormones and produce other hormones such as oestrogen and testosterone, which have healthier and more enjoyable effects.

12

What can I do?

The one good thing about gynaecological conditions is that so many of them respond to changes in lifestyle. It would be pointless – and inaccurate – to blame yourself for developing a disease, as there are too many factors involved to pick out just one. But it is wonderfully empowering to realize that there is much you can do to alleviate symptoms or even reverse their effects. While considering your options, you can improve your chance of a full cure, and reduce the risk of your problem occurring again.

Health educators recognize the value of lifestyle changes in both preventing gynaecological conditions and easing their symptoms. Stress reduction, exercise and nutrition come up again and again in medical advice – more about those in later chapters. This chapter looks at other simple, practical steps you can take right now.

Lifestyle adjustments

Knowing what caused your gynaecological condition in the first place would be useful. It's hard to say why a fibroid, for example, grew in the particular spot that made it so painful. But we do know some of the factors that make their growth more likely, as explained in Chapter 3. There's nothing we can do about some risk factors for illness, such as medical history and genetics. Fortunately, many of those that have a major effect on health are largely within our own control.

Smoking

Perhaps surprisingly, tobacco is linked with several gynaecological conditions, from painful periods to cervical cancer. Giving up smoking will not only work wonders for your complexion and your general health: it may be enough to make your dysmenorrhoea bearable. And chronic coughing is a risk factor for both uterine prolapse and urinary incontinence.

Alcohol

Drinking to excess increases your risk of many conditions, including fibroids. See Chapter 15 on nutrition for more information.

Weight

Being heavily overweight increases your risk of many diseases, including endometrial cancer. This is probably at least partly because body fat increases your oestrogen levels. However, it has other harmful effects too. Uterine prolapse, for example, is exacerbated by excess weight putting pressure on the internal organs.

Bowel health

Constipation puts pressure on prolapsed organs, and increases the pain of conditions such as dysmenorrhoea. It's a side effect of many medications, such as codeine-based painkillers. It is more likely if you eat a lot of processed food and lead a sedentary life. Constipation is easy to cure by eating plenty of fruit and vegetables, drinking more fluids and taking some exercise on most days.

Chemicals

Our environment is full of chemicals that didn't exist 50 years ago and that have never been tested for their effect on our health. Others, which have been cleared for use on our bodies, have also come under suspicion as new research uncovers possible links with disease. So it makes sense to avoid those that have any question marks over them.

It's important to wash your hands after using any chemicals – for example cleaning or gardening – before you use the loo, to avoid transferring any to your genital area. It has been suggested that using talcum powder on the perineum (the area between the vagina and anus) may increase the risk of ovarian cancer. Douching (washing inside the vagina) unbalances the body's natural self-cleansing secretions, and increases the risk of yeast infections such as thrush. And anything that damages the fragile membranes around the genital area also increases the risk of a sexually transmitted infection, as bacteria can enter through tiny scratches.

Another concern is about 'gender-bending' chemicals called xenoestrogens, which are mainly by-products of industry and agriculture. Because the structure of these pollutants is similar to that of oestrogen (though their effects are more harmful), it is believed that they can 'trick' the body into using them instead. They have been found to change the sex of male fish in polluted rivers, and they may reduce men's sperm counts. They have also been linked with oestrogen-related conditions, including cancers. Although they haven't been definitively proved to cause cancer, why take the risk?

Reducing your contact with xenoestrogens may lower your risk of developing these conditions. They are so widespread that they are hard to escape altogether, but you can reduce your exposure by avoiding:

- plastic food containers (especially in microwaves – use heat-resistant glass);
- chemical treatments for pets or gardens – and keep away from fields and golf courses when they've just been sprayed;
- harsh household chemicals, especially those with a strong smell, such as solvents;
- dry cleaning.

Sexual health

We're all now aware that unprotected intercourse – without using a condom – can lead to infection with human immunodeficiency virus (HIV), which in turn can lead on to acquired immunodeficiency syndrome (AIDS). But changes in sexual behaviour during the past 30 years have increased the risk of other sexually transmitted infections (STIs) too. These are now so widespread that some are becoming resistant to the antibiotics that had kept them in check since the mid-twentieth century.

STIs are not only dangerous in themselves. Cervical cancer and pelvic inflammatory disease (PID) are just two of the serious conditions that can arise as further effects. The damage STIs can cause to internal organs also exacerbates the effects of other gynaecological conditions.

The best defence against STIs is barrier contraception, in the form of male or female condoms. These are essential to use with a new partner, or in a non-monogamous relationship. They aren't 100 per cent guaranteed, but nothing except monogamy or celibacy provides more protection.

All sexually active women should have regular smear (Pap) tests to look out for early signs of cervical cancer. If you have numerous partners or are in a non-monogamous relationship, you should also have regular sexual-health check-ups.

Bear in mind that neither condoms nor health checks are guaranteed fail-safe. Be alert for changes such as unusual discharge or painful urination. And whether you're sexually active or not, symptoms such as pelvic pain and abnormal bleeding should never be ignored.

Learn to relax

Relaxation techniques not only make you feel better while you're doing them; their benefits continue for some time afterwards. A full-body relaxation is beneficial to several of the conditions in this book. It reduces blood pressure, for example, which is known to be linked with fibroids. It may also help to stabilize blood-sugar levels, therefore easing the symptoms of PMS. It relieves pain, especially in the back, a frequent side effect of gynaecological conditions.

Full-body relaxation

Tightening your muscles before letting go of them seems to increase the relaxation you feel. Allow yourself at least five minutes to carry out this simple but deeply effective technique.

If you're stuck somewhere sitting, you can relax much of your body using the same method. Even if you're standing, you can relax your shoulders, arms and back, which tend to hold more than their share of tension. Otherwise, put a rug or towel on the floor in a room that is comfortably warm and quiet.

Lie down on your back with feet apart and arms slightly away from the body, palms facing upwards. If pain in your back or abdomen makes lying flat uncomfortable, raise your knees to a comfortable level or put a pillow under them. Keep your feet on the floor and rest them against the wall to stop them slipping away.

Close your eyes and let your breathing slow down. Breathe out before you tense each part of your body. Breathe naturally as you feel the relaxation spreading through you. Feel tension pour out like a liquid soaking through the floor and away. Pause for a moment after relaxing each part of the body to feel this release of tension.

Starting with your left foot, clench your toes, flex the foot with toes upwards and try to tighten every muscle in the foot, lifting it slightly off the floor. Hold this for a few seconds, then relax. Then tighten the calf muscles. Hold this for a few seconds, then relax the calf. Work your way up each leg this way.

Moving your attention to your torso, pause for a moment to become aware of any pain you're holding. Instead of tightening muscles around that area if it's painful, imagine yourself breathing relaxation into it.

Continue working your way up the front of the body, tightening and releasing the muscles except in the painful areas. Then work your way up the back, then each arm.

Lift the shoulders and tense the neck as tightly as you can, raising the head slightly, then release. Clench your teeth and squeeze your face into a tight grimace. Relax with lips slightly apart.

Finally, take a few moments to feel how heavy your head is, sinking into the floor, with your whole body perfectly relaxed. Lie peacefully for a few minutes, enjoying the relaxation.

Then roll on to your side and get up slowly. On an in-breath, stretch your arms above your head and bring them slowly down to your sides with a long outward sigh.

Relieve back pain

Backache is a common symptom of many women's health conditions. Pain radiating from the uterus is frequently felt in the lower back. Conditions that distort the womb can put a strain on the ligaments holding it in place. Hormonal changes also weaken some of the muscles and ligaments supporting the complex structure of the spine. In addition, we tend to hunch protectively around a pain in the abdomen, or slump into a chair when feeling weak from heavy bleeding. These habits put pressure on the spine, exacerbating pain and cramping the internal organs.

So anything you do to strengthen and protect your back will reduce a major source of pain. Best and simplest is to improve your posture. Wearing low-heeled shoes will help, and Pilates classes are valuable. For one-to-one work, go to a practitioner of bodywork such as Feldenkreis or Alexander Technique – they specialize in relieving pain by improving posture. Meanwhile, try this simple exercise.

Perfect posture exercise

Stand in front of a full-length mirror, and check that your centre of gravity is above the middle of your feet. If your back is overarched, your pelvis will be level with or beyond your toes. If you're slumped, your shoulders will be rounded, your breasts sagging and your head either despondently bowed or lifted like a tortoise's. All these put a strain on your neck and back.

Now try to stand up straight, your weight equally distributed between both feet, feet pointing forwards, arms relaxed. Lift your shoulders and drop them a couple of times to ease the muscles. Imagine being suspended by a string from the ceiling attached to the top of your head. Try to release tension in your spine and let it find its natural curve.

Now put one hand on the front of your pelvis, the other on your tailbone. Imagining that your pelvis is a bowl of water, use your hands to find out how level it is. If you arch your back the imaginary water will pour out at the front; if you slump, it will pour out at the back. Tilt it from side to side to see if you stand with one hip higher or further forward than the other, as many of us do. Then gently try to bring your pelvis to a point where it is level.

Good posture will feel strange at first, if you've spent all your adult life wearing high heels, carrying a heavy shoulder-bag or working at a desk. But you should soon feel lighter and move more easily. Low backache should be relieved, and much of your pelvic pain may disappear.

13

Dealing with stress

Psychological factors, such as stress and how we deal with it, are now being recognized as major players in our health. When it comes to gynaecological conditions, they are more important than ever. That's because reproductive health is strongly influenced by our hormones, which in turn are influenced by our state of mind. Under stress, for example, our bodies produce excessive amounts of the hormone cortisol. This has the side effect of counteracting progesterone and therefore increasing the effects of oestrogen.

Stress is known to exacerbate many of the conditions covered in this book. But as most of them are hormone-related, it is also suspected of increasing our risk of developing them in the first place. Additionally, stress is now recognized as a major factor in chronic pain conditions, including pelvic pain. Learning to control its harmful effects on the body could help to relieve long-term pain that has not been cured by medicine or surgery and cannot be traced to a specific cause. If this is your major reason for considering hysterectomy, you may be able to bring your pain under control without the need for surgery.

Defeating all sources of pressure is beyond the scope of a book. Luckily we don't need to create an impossibly stress-free life. A much simpler answer is to change our response to pressure so that it no longer damages our health. This chapter looks at how to become stress-resistant in a frequently stressful world.

Make yourself stress-proof

Being ill, or exhausted by hormonal problems, is stressful in itself. And when you're coping with pain or heavy bleeding, it's hard to find extra energy for dealing with outside problems.

There are practical ways of reducing stress, of course. You can avoid difficult people, schedule enough time for yourself and even develop a new-found ability to say 'No'. You can work on tackling problems at their source, whether it's making time to do the exercises that relieve your pain, or ensuring you have supplies of extra-absorbent sanitary pads at work. All of these will help. But it's hard to avoid facing stressful situations at some point. The solution is more in your response to stress than in any ability to avoid it. You can't banish all stress-triggers from your life, but you can change the way you deal with them.

According to psychologists, some people are more stress-resistant than others by nature. Though it's nice to be born that way, it is also something that can be developed. Researchers have looked into the way stress-resistant people behave, and they report that anyone can practise the coping traits that allow people to shrug off pressure.

Some people are more driven to perfection than others, and get anxious if things go wrong. If that's you, work at letting things slide off. If you can't change the situation, change the way you look at it. Letting go of perfectionism is one stress-proofing factor.

We tend to think it's better to express bad feelings than to bottle them up. But is that true? Some studies show that people who simply push upsetting thoughts out of their minds are happier and more successful than those who are more tuned in to their feelings. High levels of hostility are associated with more heart attacks and a higher risk of dying from them. And it is expressing anger, rather than just feeling it, that doubles the risk.

But the psychologists aren't advising you to keep your grievances simmering on a back burner. They recommend either talking things through with the person who annoyed you or solving the problem as best you can, then getting on with your life. Rather than having to struggle with anger, ward it off with meditation or breathing exercises to soothe yourself when you're faced with an irritant.

If your short fuse is due to more than just hormonal mood swings, consider seeing a psychotherapist. A short course of something practical such as cognitive behaviour therapy can help you deal with this unhelpful trait, and many others. You can learn to be more in command of your life. Longer-term psychotherapy has proved less likely to help. But getting things off your chest with friends, that natural version of talking therapy, offers a safety valve – as long as you help each other to feel better instead of encouraging a gloomy and negative life-view.

Some other factors are equally important, researchers have found. Stress-resistant people tend to look on difficulties as challenges, and face up to them. They have well-defined personal goals. They live balanced lives that include exercise, relaxation and time off with friends and family. Other studies have found that stress-resistant people tend to be outgoing and emotionally stable. They accept commitments instead of feeling trapped by them. They tend to be easy-going and self-confident, and feel supported by their families.

You can't always choose your circumstances, but you can choose how to react to them. You can even choose your character, to some extent: pretending to feel confident actually makes you more confident. Because stress-resistant people feel in control of their lives, they don't easily sink into a feeling of helplessness that leads to anxiety and on to depression. That helpless feeling increases our perception of physical pain, making it considerably harder to bear.

Exercise plays an important part in a stress-proofing programme. It's not only proved to relieve pelvic symptoms, but is also one of the best ways of shaking off stress. That satisfying high after a good work-out lasts much longer than the sweat you've worked up. On top of that, a fit body copes better with the muscle-knotting, heart-pounding upsets we all encounter on bad-hormone days.

Stress-proofing strategies

- Don't be a perfectionist. If people don't like your cobwebs, offer them a duster!
- Learn to control your temper if you lose it easily. You really can learn to shrug off annoyances.
- Solve problems or forget them. But never let them continue to the point where you feel helpless and trapped.
- Accept your current commitments and focus on the pleasures rather than the work they cause.
- Keep up your friendships and spend time with the people you love.
- Talk things through with friends when you feel the need.
- Make a note of things that improve your self-esteem, either because you're good at them or because you feel they're valuable. Give yourself time to do them.
- If stressful thoughts come to your mind, just let them float on out. Meditation may help with this.
- Copy the behaviour of stress-resistant people: smiling, for example, actually can lift your spirits.

Make meditation part of your routine

Once thought of as faintly mystical, meditation is now almost mainstream. At its simplest, meditation is just a way of pressing 'Pause' on the hectic activity in our brains and finding a bit of space to regroup in. As well as aiding relaxation and giving your busy mind a rest, it can reduce blood pressure, ease pain and assist physical healing.

How does it work? Meditation puts your brain into a different gear, producing 'alpha' waves instead of the usual workaday 'beta' waves.

This relaxed but alert alpha state is different from dreaming (when the brain produces 'theta' waves) or sleeping deeply ('delta' waves). It sometimes happens naturally when we are deeply relaxed, soaking in a warm bath, engrossed in watching the sun set or listening to peaceful music. Meditating helps us to focus and live fully in the here and now – enjoying the present moment, letting go of health anxieties and pain.

It can be hard to settle down to meditation. The conscious mind dislikes any restriction. It reacts like a baby resisting sleep and throws up increasingly clever ruses to distract you. You can't get comfortable. You notice your heartbeat, which sounds unhealthily loud. Your everyday worries may come urgently to mind. Your mind will be filled with chatter.

Don't react to this. As thoughts enter your mind, just let them pass through without giving them your attention; you can still reach the alpha state. When, as inevitably happens, you realize your thoughts have wandered, just bring your attention back, without worrying, to the movement of breath and the phrase you're silently repeating (see below).

Before long your breath starts to slow down and it becomes easier to bring your focus back after each detour. You stop fidgeting and feel more peaceful. Soon you may start experiencing bigger benefits. If you're having PMS mood swings or bouts of pain, you may already be noticing that they don't come so often or last so long.

When you feel stressed, try to bring your mind into that meditative state for a few minutes. It should at least make it easier to cope, and you may be surprised what a powerful effect it has on the symptoms themselves. And try to make meditation a routine, doing it the same time every day and, as far as possible, in the same place.

Healing meditation

Sit comfortably on a straight-backed chair. Keeping your back straight assists the meditative process.

Set an alarm for ten minutes, so you don't keep wondering how long you've been meditating. Choose a word or short phrase to meditate on, such as 'Perfect balance', if you feel your hormones are out of balance, or 'I feel well'. Rest your hands in your lap. Close your eyes and let your breathing settle into a steady and relaxed rhythm.

Each time you breathe out, silently say the phrase and imagine a feeling of wellness spreading through you. Don't think about it more than that, just say the words with the intention of feeling well.

When you notice that your mind has wandered, don't criticize yourself. Just bring your attention back to the meditation. This happens to everyone, even experienced meditators.

Don't worry if you think you're not meditating properly. Just giving your mind a bit of thought-free space does some good. And you may not recognize the alpha state at first; it's a very subtle change.

At the end, open your eyes and sit quietly for a moment. Enjoy the peaceful, uncluttered feeling before doing anything else.

Choose one positive word or phrase, and stick to that for a week. Write in your diary that you're going to spend ten minutes every morning meditating on it. That way, you don't have to make any decisions or have anything else to distract you from doing it.

Help with meditation

There are as many meditation methods as there are reasons to meditate. Many people have learnt to meditate from books or friends or on a short course. Buddhist groups run some courses, or you could ask for information on local groups at your library.

The best-known form is Transcendental Meditation, which offers personal tuition, your own mantra – a word or phrase to repeat while meditating – and follow-up sessions. Even sceptics admit that they are more likely to persevere with something they've paid a lot of money to learn. If you've tried by yourself and found it hard to establish a routine, Transcendental Meditation could be the answer for you.

14

Exercise to help you heal

We all know that exercise is good, but it can be hard to get started at the best of times. When you're suffering from a painful condition, it's natural to feel cautious about suddenly making strenuous new demands on your body. Yet this is the time when you stand to benefit most from becoming more active.

Exercise and hormones

A mountain of research shows that the right kind of exercise can ease many gynaecological symptoms such as pelvic pain, backache, stiffness and exhaustion. It can have an instant effect on the psychological side such as mood swings, anxiety and depression.

Women's health problems are strongly connected with hormones. Exercise works on these directly, by increasing the body's output of mood-lifting chemicals called endorphins. It also affects them indirectly, by subtly regulating the production of major reproductive hormones such as oestrogen.

Studies have shown, for example, that women who take regular exercise are less likely to develop fibroids or endometrial cancer. As this is thought to be at least partly due to the effects of exercise on regulating oestrogen, it suggests that exercise could be equally good for other oestrogen-related conditions – and that's most of those in this book.

You may be experiencing menopausal symptoms, either as a result of your health condition, or because of your age, or as a side effect of medical or surgical treatment. Exercise has been proved second only to HRT in coping with symptoms of the menopause such as hot flushes – but without any of HRT's unwanted effects.

When you're not in peak health, you need something that will motivate you to continue when you're feeling under the weather. So don't start an activity just because it's said to be useful. Choose something you'll enjoy enough to feel cheated if you have to miss out. Other aids to motivation are finding a friend to exercise with, or signing on for a class you have to pay for in advance.

Accidental effects

You have special needs to consider at present. Activities that work wonders when you're in good health can make you feel worse when you're coping with a disorder. So take it gently, especially while you get started.

The pounding movement of running is likely to exacerbate pelvic pain. As energetic exercise promotes blood circulation, it can make you bleed even more during a heavy period. And heavy lifting can exacerbate a prolapse, so the last thing you want to do in that condition is to take up weight training.

Until your gynaecological condition is sorted out, you are right to be a bit cautious. You need to take special care not to make any of your symptoms worse. This chapter looks at how to be active without the risk of exacerbating your condition.

Tell your doctor

Please check with your doctor before starting any exercise programme. Your doctor will be able to say what's safe and advisable for your individual condition. There may be certain things you shouldn't try at present. On the other hand, you may even be able to take up exercise on prescription.

Also, when you're having treatment or being investigated for a health condition, your doctor needs to know about any variations. Even healthy lifestyle changes such as taking up exercise might influence the results of tests, or the effects of a treatment.

Start exercising with the help of qualified instructors, if at all possible. Your local leisure centre may have staff who are trained to deal with special needs such as your current limitations. Or your doctor may be able to refer you to specialist courses run by physiotherapists, such as therapeutic Pilates.

Target your symptoms

Exercise improves your general health, which will increase your body's ability to combat infections, inflammation and any other kind of condition. It also has a regulating effect on your hormones. Where you'll feel the immediate effect is on your symptoms. So choose a routine that's tailored to relieving those.

Back pain

Stiffness can quickly set in when pain becomes a habit. The suggestions for pelvic pain will meet your needs for aerobic exercise. And free up your back with gentle exercises aimed at loosening pain-knotted muscles. These include:

- stretches
- gentle forms of yoga with an instructor who knows how to look after your back
- Pilates.

Exhaustion

It's hard to summon up the energy to take exercise when you're tired. But as long as your doctor agrees, try:

- walking in a park or other green outdoor scenery
- swimming
- t'ai chi.

Heavy bleeding

To gain the benefits of exercise without increasing blood loss, choose a non-strenuous routine that will work your muscles and increase flexibility. Anything slow-moving is suitable, and a rhythmic movement also helps. Try:

- yoga
- resistance exercise
- qi gong.

Pelvic pain

When pain is caused by congestion or dysmenorrhoea, aerobic exercise helps by stimulating blood circulation. However, high-impact movements have a painful jarring effect. So choose a low-impact, high-energy activity such as:

- brisk walking
- dancing
- aqua aerobics.

Pelvic pressure

Feelings of pressure can be caused by uterine prolapse or by some other conditions such as fibroids. (It can also be a warning sign of ovarian cancer, so go to your doctor if your condition hasn't had a definite diagnosis.) Try the following:

- One-to-one Pilates, if you can find a practitioner who is qualified to work with your condition. Pilates aims to strengthen the body's 'core' muscles, but ordinary classes may put yours under too much pressure.
- Kegel exercises, which were devised to strengthen the pelvic floor.
- Mula bandha, a yoga exercise for the pelvic floor.

PMS symptoms

The anxiety, irritation and depression caused by PMS all respond to high-energy exercise. Choose anything that will increase your body's production of feel-good endorphins, such as:

- salsa dancing
- running
- skipping.

Pelvic floor exercises

These are valuable as a preventive measure. As you already have a gynaecological condition, check with your doctor that these will not cause too much strain. If you have a prolapsed womb, for example, it's best to learn these from a specialist physio who can ensure you are not causing harm.

Kegel exercises

1 To get an idea of the muscles you need to work on, stop the flow while you are urinating, then let it start again and stop it again. Don't do this as an exercise, because it can irritate the bladder – only do it if you need to re-check that these are the muscles you're exercising.
2 Hold in your anal muscles as if stopping yourself passing wind. Release and tighten again to get the feel of this set of muscles.
3 Put a finger flat on the perineum (the skin between the vagina and the anus) and squeeze your muscles as if stopping yourself urinating. Then tighten muscles as if to stop yourself passing wind. Try to feel the pelvic floor lifting itself a tiny distance up, towards your head. Your finger should feel the tiny lifting movement inside.
4 Ensure that you're lifting muscles in and up. Rest a hand on your lower abdomen: if this pushes against your hand when you make the effort, you're straining downwards instead.
5 Make sure you're not using other muscles. Relax your buttocks, thighs and abdominal muscles. Don't hold your breath.
6 Hold the lift for four seconds, relax for four seconds, and repeat

10 or 15 times. Work up gradually to holding for ten seconds at a time.

7 Do the exercises for at least five minutes, three times a day, preferably in different positions: lying, sitting and standing.

Yoga mula bandha

1 Sit with your legs crossed. If possible, rest one heel in your groin against your perineum, which is the area between vagina and anus.
2 Try to stop an imaginary flow of urine in midstream by tightening the muscles of the pelvic floor: your mula, or root. You may be able to feel the movement with your foot. If your anus or buttocks also tighten, let them relax.
3 Practise until you feel you've got the right muscles; you should feel a very small lifting movement.
4 Breathe normally, and focus on your breath. Then, on an in-breath, lift and hold the pelvic floor for a count of five.
5 Release on an out-breath to the count of five. Repeat 6 to 12 times.

Choose the right shoes

This is surprisingly important, especially when you have a gynaecological condition. A jarring movement or a fall can cause internal pain. So choose the right shoes to reduce the risk of falls, stabilize the feet and protect your aching back.

Different shoes are made for different activities because your foot and leg movements vary. Running, for example, is a forward-only motion, so running shoes are extremely flexible, have good traction on the soles to prevent slipping, but provide little support for sideways movement. Fitness shoes are made for aerobics, combining flexibility, support and cushioning to reduce the risk of impact injuries.

Cross-trainers are a compromise, aimed at suiting quite a range of activities. A good pair should be enough when you're starting out. But they're not really flexible enough for running, as they'll make your feet and your leg muscles work harder to bend the foot with each step. And if you move on to advanced levels in any activity, you may find you need more specialized footwear to avoid injuries.

As well as being right for the activity you're planning to do, your shoes should meet your individual needs. More cushioning means less stability, for example. You may need more cushioning if your arches aren't springy enough to protect your joints from impact, or more stability (such as high-tops) if you turn your ankle easily.

When buying shoes, shop in the afternoon, when your feet have spread to their maximum width. Check that shoes fit well, neither large enough to let your foot slide around nor small enough to pinch. Sports shoes should feel firm but comfortable. You shouldn't have to break them in, but when they become as comfy as slippers they're not supporting your feet any more.

Protect your back

Back pain is a common symptom of gynaecological disorders, and exercise is an excellent way of relieving it. However, it's easy to exacerbate the pain if you make the wrong moves. This is more likely to happen when you're exercising alone or with an unqualified instructor. Try starting out in a class or with a trainer.

Pilates can be good for your back, as it includes many controlled movements that don't put a strain on the spine. If you're in a class, though, watch out for any moves that are too advanced. Aerobic and resistance exercises also help, by improving oxygen supply and strengthening the muscles to support the spine more securely.

Stretching, yoga and aerobic exercise can ease backache and increase flexibility, so that you become less likely to put your back out. But take care that overenthusiastic or under-qualified yoga teachers don't encourage you to make painful moves. Look for teachers registered with major organizations such as the British Wheel of Yoga or Yoga Biomedical Trust. Don't do anything that doesn't feel safe to you.

Not all kinds of exercise are suitable. Cycling, for example, frequently causes lower back pain. Adjusting the saddle may help. If not, try adjusting the handlebars or experimenting with different shapes of bike. But if the pain persists, maybe you should swap to a different kind of exercise.

It is important to be aware of your posture when you're exercising, being especially careful not to either slump or arch your lower back. Building strength in your abdominal muscles helps to hold everything in place.

RICE for injuries

If you pull a muscle or hurt a joint, taking immediate action can prevent long-term damage. You need RICE:

- Rest – stop what you're doing at once and sit or lie down.
- Ice – put a cold pack on the injured spot as quickly as possible, especially if it starts swelling, and keep it there for 15 to 20 minutes. A

packet of frozen peas will do. If you're using ice cubes, put a thin cloth between them and your skin to prevent frostbite.

- Compression – an elastic bandage may help to keep the swelling down, but don't use anything tight enough to restrict the blood supply.
- Elevation – raise the injured part as often as possible to help it drain. If it's your leg or knee, prop it up on cushions rather than putting your foot on a chair, to support your knee joint.

For a pulled muscle, repeat the ice treatment at least four times a day until the swelling has disappeared. Take gentle exercise to keep the muscle mobile as it heals. While you're recovering, do some balance exercises to help your body relearn its old skills.

If anything other than a muscle is injured – a twisted knee, for example – get it checked by a GP as it may need treatment. Rest a non-muscle injury as much as possible and protect it from further damage. If you're bleeding, clean the injury, put on antiseptic and cover it. Ibuprofen is recommended as a painkiller directly after an injury, since aspirin promotes blood flow and paracetamol doesn't relieve muscle inflammation.

These are first-aid techniques for minor injuries only. For anything serious, especially if you've hit your head or feel confused, you need an ambulance.

If you often get the same kind of injury, or keep hurting yourself during the same kind of exercise, get a specialist trainer or a sports physio to check what you're doing wrong and how to avoid it.

15
Eat to aid your hormones

The foods we eat have such a strong impact on all areas of health that it's not surprising they affect hormones too. What may be surprising is quite how much of a difference you can create by making a few simple changes to your everyday diet. Eating the right iron-rich foods, for example, will help prevent anaemia caused by heavy bleeding.

There has been a lot of research into the effect of food on gynaecological conditions. Although it comes from different angles, much of it converges on one point: it's largely to do with oestrogen. It seems that the food you eat may increase or reduce the amount of oestrogen in your body. In addition, certain foods contain compounds similar enough to oestrogen to trick your body into using these 'phytoestrogens' instead.

Oestrogen is the common factor in many of the conditions for which you might be considering a hysterectomy. Although oestrogen is essential throughout our reproductive lives, and continues to play a helpful role even after the menopause, too much of it can be harmful. Oestrogen is what fuels many of the most aggressive cancers, including those of ovaries and womb. It also promotes the development of endometriosis, fibroids, polyps and other troublesome growths in and around the uterus. It makes sense, then, that a diet reducing the amount of excess oestrogen in your body could reduce your risk of developing these problems, and slow down their growth if you already have them.

Meaty questions

Scientists have found that women who eat a high-fat diet, including a lot of red meat, are twice as likely to develop fibroids, for example, as vegetarians eating a lot of natural fibre. That seems to be because a meaty, fatty diet encourages the body to produce more oestrogen.

It's not certain why cutting down on meat helps. North American sources point out that factory-farmed meat is full of artificial hormones similar to oestrogen. These make the animals put on weight quickly and cheaply, but also increase oestrogen levels in the people who eat them. Most meat sold in the United States has been raised on industrial farms, where it may have been fed on genetically modified grains, injected with growth hormones and given other drugs.

However, growth hormones have been banned in the UK and the rest of the European Union since the 1980s. Could they still be affecting women who ate them, perhaps as children more than 20 years ago? It's possible, as their effects on a child's developing body may be stronger than on an adult's. It's also possible that we may eat more of them than we think. Some imported meats have been found to contain banned substances. And because much cheap meat comes from outside the EU, you've no idea of the conditions under which it was raised.

In the UK, meat in packaging showing the red tractor logo is guaranteed by the National Farmers' Union to meet all legal requirements. Safest of all is organic meat, which has never been allowed to contain hormones, antibiotics or any other residues of chemical farming practices.

A related point is that much red meat – especially cheap cuts, and the kind found in processed foods – is high in saturated fat. And a high-fat diet in itself seems to increase the risk of oestrogen-fuelled disease. It also makes us put on weight, another risk factor for fibroids and oestrogen-dependent cancers.

Chicken is often touted as a cheap, low-fat alternative to red meat. However, like other meat, chicken imported from outside the EU has been found to contain chemical residues including hormones. And factory-farmed chicken – by far the commonest kind – is a major source of food-poisoning bacteria. Not a healthy alternative, even if low in fat. So again, organic is the safest option.

Eating a lot of meat and dairy produce may also increase the body's production of prostaglandins, which cause the intense pain and nausea of dysmenorrhoea and endometriosis.

Vegetable benefits

Vegetarian diets, proved to reduce the risk of fibroids, are usually full of fruit and vegetables. These are packed with all kinds of valuable nutrients. But perhaps most importantly, they are rich in fibre, which seems to help the body to excrete excessive oestrogen.

Leafy greens and cruciferous vegetables, such as cabbage and broccoli, seem particularly useful. As well as combating excess oestrogen, they are unusually rich in nutrients that help the immune system fight illness.

Weight of evidence

As well as eating healthy foods, it's important to keep to a healthy weight. Being underweight puts pressure on your reproductive system, which can't function if you don't have enough body fat. But being heavily overweight exacerbates many gynaecological conditions. It increases your body's production of oestrogen, in an unhealthy form. It cramps your internal organs at a time when they may already be coping with other pressures. And it is often a sign that you're eating unwholesome junk foods.

If you need to lose weight, don't go on fad diets. These never work but leave you feeling worse. Just substitute snacks and ready meals with the revitalizing foods listed in this chapter.

The phytoestrogen conundrum

Some of the research into food and hormones seems contradictory. Take phytoestrogens, for example – the oestrogen-like compounds contained in certain foods. There are two main kinds: isoflavones, most famously found in soy beans, and lignans, abundant in seeds and nuts and their oils.

They are of interest to women with oestrogen-related illness, as there is a possibility that phytoestrogens may protect against the hormone-disrupting effects of xenoestrogens – industrial pollutants that trick their way into the body by mimicking oestrogen. Though this hasn't yet been proved, the theory is that phytoestrogens may be able to mimic oestrogen more successfully, denying the xenoestrogens a chance to enter the body and affect the hormones.

However, phytoestrogens are more famous for helping women through the perimenopause by boosting their declining levels of oestrogen. That seems to be backed up by the experience of women in China and Japan, where soy and other phytoestrogen-rich foods have been part of the everyday diet for centuries. They don't report suffering so much from menopausal symptoms, such as hot flushes, as women in the West.

So surely that would make phytoestrogens bad for women who already have too much oestrogen, or whose bodies are reacting badly to oestrogen? At first glance, the evidence suggests that could be true. One study found that women taking phytoestrogen supplements for five years or more were at increased risk of developing endometrial hyperplasia, which can lead on to cancer. Another reported that women eating a lot of soy products and suffering from oestrogen-related conditions found their symptoms eased off when they gave up soy. The researcher reported that the women's fibroids, polyps, endometriosis and severe dysmenorrhoea all improved once they were no longer being fuelled by soy products.

Yet the surprising fact is that women in China and Japan suffer less from oestrogen-related diseases than westerners, despite their high intake of phytoestrogens. That could be partly because they have traditionally been slimmer, more active and less likely to drink alcohol or smoke than women in the West. These attributes reduce their risk of many diseases, including those that are oestrogen-related. But they also eat phytoestrogens in a very different form. A traditional Japanese diet contains about 25–50mg isoflavones a day. That comes from a variety of fresh produce and traditional foods, many of them based on fermented soy.

Women in western countries are eating far more phytoestrogens than in the past. But we're eating them in novel forms, highly concentrated and without all the other phytonutrients contained in their natural plant form. Since the 1990s, there has been an explosion in the number of new soy-based products appearing on western supermarket shelves. And phytoestrogen supplements are now available containing up to 1000mg isoflavones. In addition, soy is used as a cheap filler in many processed foods. That means that if you're not cooking your own meals from fresh ingredients you may already be swallowing a lot of phytoestrogens, though not necessarily in a healthy form.

No wonder phytoestrogens may not be working so well over here. Until novel soy products and supplements have been around long enough for their long-term effects to be known, it's safest to eat phytoestrogens the traditional way. If you wish to try them, eat some tofu (bean curd), edamame beans, or fermented soy products such as miso, natto and tempeh. (Soy sauce doesn't contain enough isoflavones to count.)

Natural phytoestrogens are thought to do our hormones nothing but good. But this is not yet known for sure, so don't add any to your diet without telling your doctor. If you have had an oestrogen-dependent cancer, it's probably not worth taking the risk. Otherwise, having up to one 85g serving a day should be safe. But if your symptoms worsen, stop and let your doctor know.

Fightback foods

A healthy diet for anyone is based on vegetables and fruit, with whole grains and some high-quality protein. Some foods in particular can keep us feeling in top form when we're coping with hormonal illness.

These 'fightback foods' help us stay on top of things, mentally, physically and emotionally. They work in various ways: increasing energy, reducing stress, keeping our brains sharp or fighting off pains and infections.

They're rich in things we need during this time. Iron, for example, is the mineral we lose during heavy periods, leaving us feeling constantly tired. Zinc is an all-round useful mineral that boosts the immune system, promotes healing and may combat depression. B vitamins, especially B6, protect against stress and hormone-related mood swings. Omega-3 oils fight inflammation and pain. Plentiful supplies of vitamin C build peak health and energy. It also helps the body absorb iron to counter the draining effects of heavy bleeding. Because you're getting these nutrients in their natural form instead of concentrated in supplements, it's difficult to upset your nutritional balance and almost impossible to overdose. Filling up on these nutritious foods has an added benefit: they take the place of overprocessed products. Those not only do no good, but actively reduce the body's capacity to deal with stress, fatigue and opportunistic infections.

Here are some of the best.

- *Porridge*. Whole grains of all kinds are good for us, especially during times of hormonal upheaval. But oats are the best of the bunch. They contain a kind of fibre called betaglucan that stabilizes blood sugar levels, reducing mood swings along with the risk of diabetes. They are exceptionally valuable in protecting women from heart disease and breast cancer after menopause or hysterectomy, and are packed with nutrients that keep your immune system strong.
- *Garlic*. Among its many benefits, garlic keeps your circulation brisk, toning up the whole body and improving the blood supply to your brain. It has antiseptic qualities and also helps you digest food to make better use of the other nutrients you're eating. There's even some evidence that it might improve physical endurance, when you're suffering from fatigue. And garlic's relatives – onions, and vegetables with an oniony taste like leeks – are just slightly less concentrated sources of the same benefits.
- *Mackerel*. A rich source of anti-inflammatory nutrients. Along with other oily fish like wild salmon and sardines, herring and fresh (not tinned) tuna, it provides the omega-3 oils that counteract inflammation – source of much pelvic pain. On top of that, mackerel adds B vitamins and magnesium to counteract stress.
- *Bananas* are packed with potassium and vitamin B6 to reduce feelings of stress and soothe mood swings. If you're in a hurry, a

banana's a ready-packed breakfast to eat on the train; if you also grabbed something less healthy a banana will calm your indigestion. And as an evening snack, a banana will help you sleep.

- *Ginger.* Like garlic, this is another all-round worker. It eases muscle pain by improving blood circulation and keeps the immune system strong. It reduces the incidence of headaches, migraines, indigestion and nausea – a common side effect of some hormonal drugs. It can ease period pains and backache too.
- *Berries.* All black and red berries are packed with vitamin C and infection-fighting compounds. Cranberry juice has been proved to relieve urinary infections such as cystitis by stopping bacteria sticking to the bladder wall.
- *Green leafy vegetables.* Spinach, kale, spring greens, chard – they're ideal foods for when you're coping with gynaecological conditions. They provide vitamin E to ease menstrual symptoms, vitamin K to strengthen your bones against the weakening effect of certain drugs, potassium to soothe anxiety, vitamin C to bolster your immune system and the antioxidant beta carotene to protect your cells from damage. And there's hardly a calorie in the whole lot.
- *Nuts and seeds.* High in fat but also in a whole string of nutrients, these make a satisfying nibble when you can't fight off a snack attack. The vitamin B6, magnesium and vitamin E in nuts combat the PMS-like symptoms and bloating effects of hormonal fluctuations. Walnuts are packed with omega-3 oils, to fight inflammation.
- *Organic meat.* Eating meat is the easy way to keep up your levels of protein, iron and zinc – all important, especially if you're having heavy periods and need to replace the lost blood. Keep it lean and don't eat it more than once a day: in the long term too much meat is harmful. Free from any risk of antibiotic residues, illegal hormones or mad-cow disease, organic meat comes from animals reared under humane and healthy conditions.
- *Sea vegetables.* A much better name than 'seaweed' for a tasty food, which could be one of Japanese women's secret defences against hormonal problems. Packed with nutrients including almost every mineral the body needs, sea vegetables provide a good supply of magnesium to reduce stress and promote healthy sleep. They even contain a little vitamin B12, hard to get from vegetarian sources. Other compounds have been shown to counteract inflammation, which may help ease the symptoms of PID. They also contain some phytoestrogens in the form of lignans.

Nutritional deficiencies

It's difficult to keep up a healthy diet when you're tired and unwell. But hardly anything you do makes more of a difference to your ability to heal. Eating whole foods is better than taking supplements, and doesn't put you at risk of making yourself worse by taking the wrong thing or causing a nutritional imbalance.

Shortage of iron is very common among women who menstruate, and heavy periods can bring you dangerously close to anaemia. The best-known sign of anaemia is tiredness. But it can also have surprisingly strong effects on both your intellect and your emotions. Slow thinking and confusion can stem from something as simple as a need for more iron in your diet.

If you're getting mood swings or other PMS-like symptoms, you may be short of B vitamins and magnesium. If you're finding it hard to concentrate or remember things, you may be short of B vitamins and omega-3 oils. Eating foods rich in these could help bring back your edge. Don't expect miracle-drug effects – even 'miracle drugs' rarely deliver these! But they could support brain function when it's under stress.

Low blood sugar can cause exhaustion, confusion and mood swings. Most people can avoid this by eating three meals a day. But as with hormonal issues, some people's bodies are more sensitive to certain changes. If you often get those symptoms but find that eating relieves them, think about changing your eating habits in order to prevent them. It could just be a question of eating smaller meals more often, or cutting out sweet foods that raise and lower blood sugar too abruptly, or eating foods that sustain you for longer. You should also get your GP to check you're not developing diabetes.

Iron vs. oestrogen control

If you suffer from heavy bleeding, you need plenty of iron-rich food to prevent anaemia. Your body absorbs iron most readily from meat, fish and eggs. But to keep oestrogen levels under control, you don't want to eat too much of those. It's hard to get enough iron from vegetable sources, unless you've been a vegetarian so long that your body has adjusted. The best compromise is to go for oily fish, which has the added benefit of counteracting pain and inflammation.

To maximize iron intake you need vitamin C, so eat iron-rich foods with vegetables and salads or a glass of orange juice. Don't drink tea or coffee within an hour of eating, as these reduce the amount of iron you absorb. And avoid bran, which can move food through your body too quickly for you to absorb the nutrients.

Should I be drinking more water?

Do we really need to drink the 2–2.5 litres – eight to ten glasses – of pure water a day, which we're often told is necessary to avoid dehydration? And is it true that by the time you feel thirsty you're already dehydrated? And that tea and coffee don't count, as caffeine's diuretic effects make us urinate more and therefore become even more dehydrated?

Many women with hormonal problems find that they retain fluid more than in the past. Drinking two litres of water a day would not only be difficult, but would leave some of us looking like balloons.

It's true that our bodies are 70 per cent water, and we lose at least two litres of fluid a day. But we take in just over a litre from the food we eat, on a typical diet. Another litre or so comes from drinks. The body tops this up with about 250ml produced by metabolic processes. Thirst will normally tell you when you need a drink, so – except in unusually hot or strenuous conditions – you're rarely at risk of dehydration unless you're ignoring your body's signals.

It's actually possible to drink too much water. If you drink much more than you need, you can over-dilute your blood so that sodium levels fall dangerously low. Although this is highly dangerous, it's also unlikely: you would have to force yourself to drink that much water.

Some health conditions such as urinary tract infections do require people to drink more water. If urinary incontinence is a side effect of your gynaecological problem, don't cut down your intake of fluids – that can lead to other problems.

Water is certainly healthier than many other drinks. Soft drinks are packed with sugar or artificial sweeteners and other additives. Fizzy drinks can irritate the bladder, exacerbating incontinence, and may play a role in reducing bone density.

But you don't have to ignore all other fluids. Tea not only doesn't cause dehydration, it is good for you. Even everyday tea is good for women with hormonal problems, as it provides compounds that relieve stress and keep the brain sharp. Green tea offers even more health benefits. And though coffee can have a diuretic effect, regular drinkers adapt to some extent. Fruit juice is healthy, and is even more refreshing if you dilute with water. One glass of fruit juice a day is enough if you're watching your weight, as it contains natural sugars. Vegetable juices are even better, as juicing gets the goodness out of a big pile into an easy-to-drink glassful. Fresh carrot juice, for example, supplies a whole shopping list of health-enhancing compounds while protecting your liver. And, unlike fruit juices, they're low in sugar. Buy a juicer to enjoy the freshest and tastiest juices in any combination you like.

You can also rehydrate with foods that are mainly water and vitamins: fruits, salads and juicy vegetables. One medium-sized orange, for example, is worth half a glass of water.

Or less alcohol?

Women are drinking more alcohol these days than ever before, and the effects are starting to show up on statistics for liver disease and cancers. It also plays a role in gynaecological conditions by increasing the harmful effects of oestrogen: one study found that women who drank beer every day doubled their risk of fibroids.

Unfair though it is, women's bodies cope less effectively with alcohol than men's do to start with. That's partly because we process the alcohol slightly differently and partly because women's bodies contain less water than men's, making the alcohol-induced dehydration so much worse the next day. And it takes more of a toll as we get older. Its dehydrating effects kick in after just two or three units, and the alcohol lingers long after the fluid has left your body.

We're advised to drink no more than two or three units a day, with at least one alcohol-free day a week. Six units counts as binge-drinking. But it's surprisingly easy to reach that number, especially with that feminine favourite, a glass of wine.

One problem is that the alcohol content of many drinks is much higher now than when we first heard of the unit system some 20 years ago. In those days a glass of wine, a measure of spirits or half a pint of beer all equalled one unit, which in the UK is equivalent to 10ml of pure alcohol. Wine was served in 125ml glasses, and was about 8 per cent alcohol by volume (AbV). Beer was up to 4 per cent AbV and spirits about 40 per cent.

Spirits and some beers have remained the same, though many beers and lagers have become stronger. A half pint of strong beer such as Stella Artois is nearer two units than one, and a 440ml can of Carlsberg Special Brew, 9 per cent AbV, is four units.

But the big difference is in wine. Today, wine bars and restaurants tend to use larger, more profitable glasses holding 175ml or even 250ml. And the wine is likely to be 12.5 per cent AbV or even stronger. So ask for 'a glass of wine' and you may well receive a 250ml glass of

14 per cent AbV wine, a full 3.5 units. So without any intention of drinking more, you've gone over the limit with just one glass.

On the other hand, some research suggests that moderate drinking – up to two units a day for women – can be good for your health. People who drink alcohol tend to live longer and be healthier on various scores, including diabetes, than teetotallers. Most of the benefits seem to stem from alcohol's stress-relieving effects and the antioxidants in wine. Red wine contains the most of these and is most strongly linked with health benefits, especially for the heart. But all the benefits are outweighed by the damage caused if you routinely drink more than two units a day.

In a nutshell

The best foods to base your diet on are vegetables of all kinds, some even more useful against certain conditions. Fruit, oily fish and cereals are next in importance. Don't stint on drinking anything other than alcohol and fizzy drinks.

Cut down on meat, to help reduce excess oestrogen, which is known to exacerbate most of the conditions in this book; North American meat is extra-oestrogenic as it may contain growth-hormone residues.

Cutting down on meat and dairy foods may also ease the pain and nausea of dysmenorrhoea and endometriosis, by reducing prostaglandin production.

Highly processed foods of all kinds seem to reduce the body's ability to fight off pain and infection.

Eat plenty of fibre-rich fruit and veg, to help control oestrogen levels and meet the added demands caused by your condition. Especially:

- For vitamin B1 (proved to ease period pains): asparagus, lettuce, mushrooms, spinach, tuna, peas, tomatoes, aubergines and Brussels sprouts.
- For vitamin B6 (to level out mood swings): spinach, peppers (capsicums), garlic, tuna, cauliflower, bananas.
- For magnesium (to relieve PMS and dysmenorrhoea): dark-green leafy vegetables, broccoli, pumpkin seeds, courgettes.
- For beta carotene (if you have heavy periods): carrots, sweet potatoes and green leafy vegetables.
- For omega-3 oils to counteract pain and inflammation: oily fish (such as salmon, mackerel and fresh tuna), flax seeds, walnuts, cauliflower, cabbage, tofu, green leafy vegetables.

Target your condition

- *Dysmenorrhoea.* Foods rich in vitamin B1 and magnesium have been proved to relieve period pain. Omega-3 oils also help. Cut down on fatty food and eat plenty of fresh fruit and vegetables, which may help to control hormone metabolism.
- *Endometriosis.* More omega-3 oils, less meat and dairy.
- *Fibroids, polyps, adenomyosis.* Cut down on meat and eat as much fruit and vegetables as you can per day – fresh if possible.
- *Heavy periods.* Plenty of iron and beta carotene.
- *PID.* Plenty of anti-inflammatory foods such as oily fish.
- *Premenstrual syndrome (PMS).* Ease your irritation and mood swings with foods rich in vitamin B6 and magnesium. Eat regularly, as low blood sugar exacerbates mood swings.

16

Menopause and HRT

The possibility of menopause is something to keep in mind if you're thinking of having any of the operations described in this book, especially a hysterectomy. If your ovaries are removed, menopause will start immediately. But even if you keep your ovaries, a hysterectomy is likely to bring on the menopause sooner than if you still had your uterus in place.

Life-saving cancer treatments can also bring the menopause on early, even if you haven't had your womb or ovaries removed. Both chemotherapy and radiotherapy can cause the ovaries to stop functioning, not necessarily at once but within the next few years. Some alternative procedures, too, may damage the complex system that keeps your ovaries working – though this is much less likely. And some of the medicines taken to control gynaecological conditions can produce side effects very similar to symptoms of the menopause.

This chapter looks at how to tell if the changes leading to menopause have started; what to do if you still want to have children; and how to cope with any symptoms.

When menopause comes early

The average age for a woman to have her last period is 51: the date of that final period is the menopause. The time of changes – usually a few years – leading up to that and shortly afterwards is known as the perimenopause.

If you stop having periods before the age of 40, it's known as premature menopause, or premature ovarian failure. Pelvic surgery and cancer treatments aren't the only reason for this. It happens to about one woman in 100, sometimes because of other health conditions or simply because it runs in some families. If you're 40 to 45 when your periods stop, it's just described as early menopause. This is more common than premature ovarian failure, as menopause can be brought forward by a number of factors including smoking and unhealthy eating.

Having your ovaries removed causes immediate menopause. Because it's so abrupt, this 'surgical menopause' usually causes more severe symptoms.

Your periods also stop after hysterectomy and some other procedures such as endometrial ablation, because you no longer have any womb lining to shed. But that isn't the same as menopause. Your ovaries should still be releasing an egg each month. (As there's nowhere for it to go, the tiny egg is just reabsorbed into your body.) Apart from not having periods or being able to get pregnant, your reproductive system is still functioning. So you should still be producing the hormones appropriate to your age.

Keeping your ovaries reduces the risk of premature menopause after a hysterectomy, but is not guaranteed to prevent it. Even if you keep your ovaries, you are likely to go through the menopause earlier than normal. Up to half of women experience ovarian failure within five years of having their uterus removed. This is sometimes because the ovaries can be damaged during an operation on the uterus. Even if they are not directly damaged, the operation can reduce their blood supply. And any pelvic surgery runs the risk of disrupting nerves and the many other complex networks that keep the reproductive system functioning. Any of these factors could cause the ovaries to fail sooner than usual. That's why alternative operations also run a small risk of triggering menopause, though this is very much less likely to happen.

How do you know you are going through perimenopause if you don't have periods any more? You are likely to start experiencing symptoms such as those below. These may not be serious enough to need treatment. But it's useful to know what's happening in your body, because your risk of certain age-related health conditions starts increasing after menopause.

Bear in mind that if it does happen, it's not all bad. Reaching menopause early does have some advantages. It reduces your lifetime risk of breast cancer and thrombosis. You cope with any symptoms at an age when you're younger and fitter than most. And if the treatments you've had haven't cured your gynaecological condition, menopause may put an end to it.

Give your ovaries their best chance

Although you can't undo any damage that's been done to the ovaries, you can ease additional pressure on them. Women who haven't had gynaecological problems may also have an early menopause, partly for lifestyle reasons. Taking up some healthier habits will maximize your ovaries' ability to keep functioning.

- Don't smoke. Smokers reach menopause on average two years early.
- Stay a healthy weight. Strict dieting, or being underweight, can stop the ovaries working. But being very overweight can also impair their function.
- Drink less than two units of alcohol a day, on average. That's one medium-sized (175ml) glass of medium-strength wine. Have a few alcohol-free days a week, too.
- Try to avoid feeling stressed. Stress can wreak havoc on your reproductive system. You can't always escape stressful situations, but you can learn how to shrug off the bad effects (see Chapter 13).

Planning for a baby?

If you've had alternative treatment because you still want to have children, it's a good idea to start trying sooner rather than later. That's true whether or not an operation has triggered the perimenopause.

Your underlying condition may mean you need to seek specialist treatment to become pregnant, and this has more chance of success the younger you are when you start. As you will probably have to join a waiting list for fertility treatment in the UK, you may want to consider private treatment. Speak first to your own doctor, who should be able to offer useful advice.

Warning signs

It's worth staying aware of changes that might be early signs of perimenopause. These aren't necessarily those that everyone associates with menopause. In the early stages, you may encounter less recognizable signs.

Menstrual changes, hot flushes and night sweats are the most likely to mean perimenopause. But do check with your doctor, as these could also be caused by your gynaecological condition or by a medicine you're taking.

- *Menstrual changes*. If you still have your uterus, your periods may become irregular, lighter or possibly heavier as you approach the menopause. But don't rely on this, as you can be in perimenopause for a long time with regular periods. If you've had a hysterectomy or endometrial ablation, you no longer menstruate, so you won't have this common warning sign.
- *Vasomotor symptoms*. These are hot flushes and night sweats, the best known signs of the perimenopause. But again, this isn't an infallible

indicator. Many women don't encounter these until late in the process, if at all. Also, check that they're not a drug side effect.

- *PMS-like symptoms*. Anyone who has suffered premenstrual syndrome (PMS) just before a period will recognize signs such as mood swings, depression, food cravings, breast swelling, fluid retention, stomach upsets, headaches or sensitivity to pain. As these are signs of hormonal upheaval, they may mean the perimenopause is getting under way. That's especially likely if you start experiencing these pre-period symptoms in your thirties or later, when you hadn't previously had much sign of PMS. Perimenopause is also likely if the symptoms erupt at random times of the month instead of just before a period, or if you're having them after a hysterectomy.

- *Loss of libido*. As the ovaries also produce testosterone, which aids sexual arousal, a loss of sex drive could be an early sign that ovaries aren't fully functioning any more. However, many women report a loss of sex drive after a hysterectomy regardless of whether they have entered perimenopause.

- *Brain and central nervous system effects*. Many women have feared they're seeing the first signs of dementia when they become clumsy, forgetful or tongue-tied. But up until your mid-fifties, it's far more likely to be a sign of perimenopausal changes in hormone levels.

- *Insomnia*. Sleepless nights are, for many women, the most unwelcome and unexpected sign of perimenopause. Surprisingly, one of oestrogen's many functions is in helping us sleep. Many other factors, from worry to an overheated bedroom, can keep us awake. But if you can't see any reason for your newfound insomnia, consider your hormones.

- *Vaginal dryness*. This can make sex uncomfortable and also increases your risk of infections such as thrush or cystitis, or of itching or general discomfort. It's usually a classic sign of perimenopause, when it results from low oestrogen levels. But that's not necessarily the case if you've had pelvic surgery, especially if it was carried out vaginally. A tiny amount of damage to the area may be enough to stop the lubricating glands functioning properly. So this may or may not be a sign that perimenopause has started.

Getting a diagnosis

If anything leads you to suspect you are entering perimenopause, check with your doctor. It's good to do some research for yourself, and it's worth asking questions and letting the doctor know your concerns. But any of the symptoms above could also mean something that's not related to the perimenopause nor even to your original gynaecological condition. As with any symptoms that cause concern, or any unexpected change in your body – see your doctor, in case it's something serious that needs prompt treatment.

You may be offered hormone tests to see if you're perimenopausal. Your hormone levels can be tested in either blood or saliva, with the proviso that neither test is 100 per cent reliable. Levels of follicle-stimulating hormone (FSH) rise during the perimenopause. Levels of oestradiol – the main form of oestrogen – fall. Therefore, in theory, tests can tell if you're approaching the menopause.

However, your levels of reproductive hormones can vary widely from one hour to the next. To gain any useful information, you need to take at least two tests a month apart. They should be done on the third day of your period, if you still menstruate. Consistently high levels of FSH and low levels of oestradiol would suggest that you have started the perimenopause.

But do listen to your body. If your hormone tests give normal results but you are having perimenopausal symptoms, remember that hormone tests can give false reassurance. Your doctor may also do a thyroid test, as many symptoms of thyroid malfunction overlap with those of the perimenopause.

What to do

There's no way of stopping the perimenopausal process once it has started. But, whether you take medicines or not, there's a vast range of self-help options that can ease the transition. Hormone replacement therapy (HRT) is the best-known medical answer to perimenopause (see below). But it isn't the only option doctors can offer.

A synthetic steroid drug called tibolone mimics the effects of other hormones as well as oestrogen, so some women find it helpful. Like oestrogen, it raises the risk of endometrial cancer, but it could be helpful after hysterectomy as you no longer have to worry about your uterus.

Disruptive hot flushes may be eased by drugs developed for other conditions, including selective serotonin re-uptake inhibitors (SSRIs, for treating depression), clonidine (blood pressure) and gabapentin (epilepsy). However, all of these have serious side effects.

There are long-term factors to consider as well as any perimenopausal symptoms. If you're going through menopause before the age of 40 and are not taking HRT or tibolone, you do face a higher than average risk of osteoporosis and heart disease. There are drugs that are claimed to protect your bones from osteoporosis, but these have serious side effects and have not been proved effective. The common drugs aimed at reducing the risk of heart disease have better statistics in their favour. These may be worth considering, especially if you're at risk for other reasons, for example because close relatives have heart disease.

However, most doctors are reluctant to put you on such drugs if you're considered 'at risk' rather than actually having signs of disease. They are more likely these days to recommend lifestyle changes than to pick up their prescription pad. A healthy diet and plenty of exercise is by far your best protection against heart disease, and a safer option than osteoporosis drugs.

Hormone replacement therapy (HRT)

In the past, prescribing oestrogen to women whose own levels were low seemed a simple answer to the symptoms of perimenopause and possibly even to the ills of ageing. The situation is now known to be much more complicated. HRT can relieve some of the signs of hormonal upheaval. But its advantages have to be balanced against its now well-known risks.

Replacement oestrogen increases the risk of endometrial cancer so steeply that if you still have your womb you will only be offered combined HRT: oestrogen balanced by progestogen. HRT also increases the risk of thrombosis (blood clots), strokes, gall-bladder disease and cancers of the breast and ovary. If you've already had a hormone-related cancer, you may be advised not to use HRT at all. And like any drug it has side effects, such as headaches, thrush and PMS-like symptoms.

On the plus side, it reduces the risk of bowel cancer and osteoporosis. Of more immediate concern to most women, HRT can ease some of the worst effects of perimenopause: the vasomotor symptoms (hot flushes and night sweats) and urogenital problems such as vaginal dryness and urinary infections. Those are the only symptoms for which HRT has been proved effective by medical research, although some women also say it has helped with others such as insomnia.

For women going through a natural menopause, doctors advise taking HRT for no more than about two years. They only recommend it to those having a particularly bad time with vasomotor and urogenital symptoms. Most women reaching a natural menopause never try HRT, and of those who do, most give it up within a year. That's not because of the health risks – the same was true before they were known. It's because very few women find the symptoms unbearable, and those who do try HRT are often put off by the side effects.

HRT and you, now

If your perimenopause has started before your mid-forties, your needs are different from those of women reaching a natural menopause. A woman's risk of many health problems increases sharply after the menopause. Reaching menopause early brings those risks forwards.

Can HRT counteract the harm done by premature menopause? Large studies have shown that, in general, it's not worth taking HRT in order to try to prevent the diseases of old age; the risks outweigh any potential benefit. It's been reported that HRT doesn't reduce the risk of heart disease, for example, and may even increase it. On the other hand, most of the heart-disease research has been done on women over 50, who started taking HRT after the menopause. Some evidence suggests that the results would be better in younger women.

Menopause has a drying effect on your skin and other tissues. Its effects on the urogenital system include making the vagina shorter, dryer and less elastic. This leads to painful sex and increases the risk of urinary infections, which can damage the kidneys, and bladder weakness, which can lead to incontinence. HRT plays a welcome role in countering these changes. For those reasons, women in premature menopause are often advised to take HRT until the time when their natural menopause would have occurred. It's certainly worth a try if you want to and if it's suitable for you. It may have more to offer if you're under 40, when a natural menopause would be a long way off. Even so, you have to weigh the increased risk of HRT-related problems against any possible benefits.

If you've had a hysterectomy or oophorectomy because of cancer, you should talk through all the implications of HRT very carefully with your doctor. If oestrogen caused your disease, the last thing you want is to put more into your body. The same is true to a lesser extent if you're suffering from any oestrogen-fuelled disorder. In favour of HRT, the dose can be controlled.

If you have had a hysterectomy for other reasons than cancer, you could ask your doctor about taking oestrogen alone. Without your uterus in place, oestrogen may no longer cause you health problems, and it doesn't have so many side effects as combined HRT.

If you're going through premature ovarian failure without having had a hysterectomy, it's worth considering combined HRT or oestrogen cream if you're suffering badly from vasomotor or urogenital symptoms.

How to take HRT

If you are having perimenopausal symptoms but are still having periods, your doctor may prescribe combined HRT patches or tablets. If your periods are irregular, this is likely to be tricyclic HRT, in which you have a bleed only once every three months. Otherwise, with cyclic HRT, you'll have a monthly bleed. As when you're taking the contraceptive Pill, HRT bleeding isn't a real period but a gap between tablets in order to let your body slough off the womb lining.

If your periods have stopped, but you haven't had a hysterectomy, you're likely to be prescribed continuous combined HRT patches or tablets. This way you don't have any bleeding at all.

If you've had a hysterectomy, your GP may prescribe oestrogen patches or tablets. You don't need progestogen as you have no uterus to protect.

Even if you still have your womb, you can protect your vagina and bladder by using an oestrogen cream on the genital area. This can be prescribed at a low enough dose not to affect other parts of the body. This solution is used by some women who don't want to use full-scale HRT. If you've had oestrogen-related problems before, you'll need to keep having regular check-ups.

HRT is available in many different formulations and dosages. If you wish to use it but the one you're prescribed causes side effects, you have several options. If the side effects are minor, keep taking the HRT for a few months to see if they ease off, as they often do within this time. If they don't, you should then ask your doctor to change the prescription. If they are major (see below), get medical help at once.

Danger signals

You should seek treatment without delay if you have any of the following symptoms. They can be signs of a serious condition that needs immediate treatment. These can happen to anyone, but are more likely if you're taking oestrogen in any form, such as HRT or the contraceptive Pill.

- Pain, redness or swelling of one leg. These may be signs of deep-vein thrombosis (DVT): a blockage in one of the large veins leading back to the heart. Go to accident and emergency (A&E), as this can be fatal. HRT often causes leg cramps, but those feel different and tend to affect both legs.
- Sudden chest pain. This is also a signal to go to A&E.
- Unusual or unexpected bleeding, for example between periods, after

hysterectomy or after your periods had stopped. Report it to your doctor, who should send you for tests.

Help yourself to a healthy menopause

Simple lifestyle changes can ease the menopausal transition so successfully that you may find you don't need HRT. Even if you do use it, self-help remedies provide a useful back-up at any age, with no side effects. For complementary and alternative therapies, see Chapter 8.

So much is now known about relieving perimenopausal symptoms that whole books are written on the subject. This is a very brief guide.

A hormone-friendly lifestyle

The lifestyle changes listed above under 'Give your ovaries their best chance' will also help you through the perimenopause. Stop smoking, drink less than two units a day of alcohol, keep to a healthy weight and learn how to shrug off stress. All of these can help to stabilize your hormones. In addition, individual symptoms can be tackled with other healthy habits.

- *Sleep well.* Many perimenopausal symptoms are related to tiredness and exacerbated by insomnia. You need seven to eight hours' restful and uninterrupted sleep a night. If you're not getting that, create a routine that will help bring it about: take some physical exercise every day, keep the last hour before bedtime for winding down, ensure the bedroom isn't overheated, put in ear plugs if necessary, go to bed eight hours before you have to get up, and set the alarm for the same time every morning.
- *Cool down.* Alleviate hot flushes by dressing in easy-to-change layers, with cardigans and zip-up body-warmers rather than sweaters that need to be pulled over your head. Carry a fan and a cool water spray for when your temperature rises.
- *Take your time.* Clumsiness and loss of balance are disturbing though temporary symptoms of the perimenopausal transition for many women. If you find you're tripping over or dropping things, slow down and give yourself a chance. Constant hurrying also exacerbates psychological symptoms such as anxiety.

Intimate care

Vaginal dryness is one of the most unwelcome signs of perimenopause, making sex painful and causing dangerous bladder infections. Unfortunately, this isn't a temporary symptom but a long-term result of low oestrogen levels. However, it is very easily treated.

If you wish to use oestrogen cream, this can be continued in the long term, but you should have regular medical check-ups. Even simpler, vaginal moisturizers are easy to use and very effective. Prescribed by your doctor or bought over the counter, they are for regular long-term use and should have no side effects (see 'Sexual recovery' section in Chapter 11 – although they are equally valuable whether you are sexually active or not).

Meditation

Meditation has a calming effect on all the emotional symptoms of perimenopause, as you might expect. By clearing the mind, it also lifts the 'brain fog' that annoys so many women at this time.

But it has surprisingly noticeable effects on physical symptoms too. Many women have found that taking a few minutes to sit quietly in meditation can actually stop a hot flush developing. There may be complex hormonal reasons for this. Or it may be because hot flushes can cause stress, which then makes the flush worse; by relieving stress, meditation breaks the vicious circle. See Chapter 13 for how to do it.

Exercise

Nothing has proved more effective than regular exercise in relieving perimenopausal symptoms without any side effects. Even hot flushes, the hardest symptom to control, can be reduced in severity as you become fitter.

Lively cardiovascular exercise – anything fast enough to increase your heart rate – strengthens your heart and lifts your spirits: try dancing, aerobics, swimming. This also helps to keep weight under control. Weight-bearing exercise such as walking builds bone strength to resist osteoporosis. Flexibility work such as yoga or stretching counteracts menopausal stiffness and pain. Eastern exercises such as t'ai chi or qi gong not only improve your balance but also have a meditative effect, relieving tension and worries.

Chapter 14 explains how to work out safely when you're suffering from a gynaecological condition. With luck, your treatment should have lifted many of those limitations. However, it's still wise to take care, especially when you're just starting out.

Nutrition

The foods you eat can alleviate or exacerbate symptoms of hormonal upheaval. So the advice in Chapter 15 will help stabilize your hormones at any time of life. Try to base your diet on vegetables, fruits, whole grains such as wholemeal bread, and some organic meat and dairy foods.

But this healthy diet has most impressive effects when you're going through the perimenopause. It is the key to avoiding symptoms such as indigestion, nausea and constipation. Importantly, it helps to prevent a particular kind of fat developing on your abdomen that has unhealthy hormonal activity and is hard to shift after menopause.

When you have passed the menopause, you need more protein and calcium than before to keep both muscles and bones strong, as your body will be using nutrients less effectively. After menopause or hysterectomy, you also need less iron than when you were losing it in monthly bleeds. Eating regular meals is important to keep blood sugar levels stable, as the risk of diabetes rises after menopause.

This is the time when phytoestrogens come into their own. Their helpfulness in oestrogen-related conditions is still being debated (see Chapter 15). But the mass of evidence in their favour is to do with combating perimenopausal and postmenopausal symptoms.

Most important, find foods you enjoy that fit into a healthy eating routine. Grimly chewing through a pile of unwanted lettuce isn't going to enhance your life, when there's a huge variety of fruit and vegetables to explore. Make time to nourish yourself in ways that you enjoy.

Glossary

Adenomyosis A condition in which an adenomyoma (tissue from the endometrium, or inner lining of the womb) grows in the myometrium, or muscle layer of the womb.

Adhesions Patches of sticky scar-like tissue, caused by endometriosis or abdominal surgery.

Bilateral salpingo-oophorectomy Removal of both ovaries and both fallopian tubes (bilateral = both sides).

Bladder The organ in which urine is stored before leaving the body via the urethra.

Cervix The neck of the uterus, which projects into the vagina.

Colpocleisis An operation to relieve a prolapse (not of the womb but of other neighbouring organs) that closes off the vagina, making sexual intercourse impossible.

Colpoperineorraphy An operation to repair the vagina after a prolapsed rectum (or small intestine) has protruded into it.

Colporrhaphy An operation to repair the vagina after a prolapsed bladder or urethra has protruded into it.

Cystitis An inflammation or infection of the bladder, in which painful urination is an early symptom.

Cystocele Prolapse of the bladder, usually caused by pelvic-floor weakness after child-bearing.

Dilation and curettage (D&C, or 'scrape') A once-common method of removing tissue from inside of the womb, either for analysis or as a treatment.

Dysmenorrhoea Painful periods.

Ectopic pregnancy A potentially life-threatening condition in which a fertilized egg implants itself somewhere other than the uterus.

Endometrial ablation Operation to remove womb lining.

Endometrial hyperplasia Thickening of the womb lining, which can lead on to cancer.

Endometriosis A condition in which tissue from the womb lining grows in other parts of the pelvis.

Endometrium The lining of the uterus, in which a fertilized egg is implanted.

Estradiol, estriol, estrone Alternative spellings for oestradiol, oestriol and oestrone, three forms of oestrogen.

Estrogen See **Oestrogen**.

Fallopian tube The tube down which an egg travels from the ovary into the uterus, and where fertilization may take place if sperm is present. There are two; one from each ovary.

Fibroid A non-cancerous growth of fibrous and muscular tissue, usually inside the uterus.

Fibroma, fibromyoma Other words for fibroid.

Hysterectomy An operation to remove the uterus, or womb.

Leiomyoma Another word for fibroid.

Menorrhagia Excessive menstrual bleeding.

Myolysis Operation to cut off blood supply to a fibroid.

Myoma Another word for fibroid.

Myoma coagulation Another name for myolysis.

Myomectomy An operation to remove fibroids.

NICE The UK National Institute for Health and Clinical Excellence – a non-government organization that provides guidelines to the National Health Service about what treatments to use on the basis of safety, effectiveness and cost. Website <www.nice.org.uk>

Oestradiol The main form of oestrogen, produced in abundance by the ovaries from puberty until menopause.

Oestriol A form of oestrogen produced during pregnancy.

Oestrogen One of the main female hormones, also linked with main gynaecological conditions. Spelt 'estrogen' in American usage.

Oestrone A form of oestrogen (weaker than oestradiol) that continues to be produced in small amounts after the menopause.

Oophorectomy Removal of one or both ovaries.

Ovaries The two organs in which eggs develop; each month, one of them releases an egg, which travels down the fallopian tube into the womb.

Pap test See **Smear test**.

Pelvic inflammatory disease (PID) Inflammation resulting from infection in one of the pelvic organs.

Pessary A pharmaceutical pessary is medicine in a form that can be inserted into the vagina like a tampon. See also Vaginal pessary.

Polyp A non-cancerous growth that may occur in several parts of the body including the uterus, and that in some cases may become cancerous.

Premenstrual syndrome (PMS) Disruptive symptoms caused by hormonal imbalance, starting shortly before a period.

Presacral neurectomy (PSN) An operation to cure pain by cutting nerves.

Proctocele Another word for rectocele.

Progestin Another word for the synthetic hormone progestogen.

Progestogen The family of hormones to which progesterone belongs; also the synthetic version of this hormone (also known as 'progestin').

Prolapse When an organ sags because the supporting tissues are weakened; uterine prolapse is often caused by child-bearing.

Radical trachelectomy An operation to remove a cancerous cervix while leaving the uterus intact.

Rectocele Prolapse of the rectum, part of the bowel.

Sacrohysteropexy An operation to support a prolapsed uterus.

Sacrospinous fixation An operation to support a prolapsed uterus.

Smear test (Pap test) A test in which a few cells are taken from the cervix, via the vagina, to check for any changes that could lead to cancer.

Ureters The two tubes that carry urine from the two kidneys to the bladder.

Urethra The tube that carries urine from the bladder out of the body.

Uterine To do with the uterus; for example, uterine cancer means a cancer of the uterus, most commonly endometrial cancer.

Uterine artery embolization (UAE) Injection of a substance into the uterine arteries to shrink fibroids.

Uterine nerve ablation (UNA) Operation to cure pain by destroying nerves in the ligament supporting the uterus.

Uterosacral ligament resection Another operation to cure pain by destroying nerves in the ligament supporting the uterus.

Uterus (womb) The organ in which the fetus grows for nine months, from the time a fertilized egg is implanted in the lining until birth.

Vagina The tube leading from the uterus out of the body.

Vaginal pessary A ring inserted into the vagina to relieve uterine prolapse.

Von Willebrand's disease An inherited disorder that causes excessive bleeding and is, therefore, one possible cause of menorrhagia.

Vulva A woman's external genitals, surrounding the opening to the vagina and including the labia.

Wertheim's hysterectomy A radical form of hysterectomy, carried out for cancer, in which lymph glands and other tissue are removed as well as the uterus, cervix, fallopian tubes and ovaries.

Womb Another word for uterus.

Useful addresses

Patients' groups are sometimes set up or funded by organizations, such as drug companies, with a financial interest. This may affect the impartiality of their advice, even though they may provide correct information. To the best of the author's knowledge, the organizations in this list are independent and open about their agenda.

UK

Cancer Counselling Trust
Edward House
2 Wakley Street
London EC1V 7LT
Tel.: 020 7843 2292
Website: www.cancercounselling.
org.uk
A charity providing free specialist counselling for those affected by cancer and their family and friends.

Cochrane Collaboration
Website: http://cochrane.co.uk
A large international non-profit group of researchers who produce independent reviews of healthcare interventions.

The Daisy Network Premature Menopause Support Group
PO Box 183
Rossendale
Lancs BB4 6WZ
Website: www.daisynetwork.org.uk
A support organization staffed entirely by volunteers. If writing to them, please enclose large s.a.e.

Drug Information Online
Website: www.drugs.com
An independent website compiled by pharmacists, providing full official information about medicines.

E-healthMD
Website: www.ehealthmd.com
A website providing information and advice, compiled by experienced health writers and backed by an international team of doctors.

Endometriosis.org
Website: www.endometriosis.org
An independent website set up by women with endometriosis. Articles are reviewed by an international team of medical experts.

Fibroid Network Online
Website: www.fibroidnetwork.com
A source of information, news and discussion groups.

Having Fun After Cancer
Website: http://after-cancer.com
Run by a cancer survivor in London, this site gives detailed information on dealing with the side effects of cancer treatment.

Hysterectomy Association
Prospect House
Peverell Avenue East
Dorchester
Dorset DT1 3WE
Tel.: 0844 3575917 (helpline)
Website: www.hysterectomy-association.org.uk
A voluntary organization set up by a patient in 1997.

National Association for Premenstrual Syndrome
421 Old Road
East Peckham
Kent TN12 5AP
Tel.: 0870 777 2178
Website: www.pms.org.uk
Part funded by complementary-healthcare companies, this is an international organization promoting the interests of women with PMS.

Natural Health Advisory Service
PO Box 117
Rottingdean
Brighton BN51 9PG
Tel.: 01273 487366
Website: www.naturalhealthas.com
Established in 1984 as the Women's Nutritional Advisory Service, this provides supplement-based nutritional treatment for symptoms of menopause and PMS.

NHS Direct
Tel.: 0845 46 47(nurse-led advice line)
Website: www.nhsdirect.nhs.uk
An excellent and easy-to-use UK government health-information resource.

Over-Count Drugs Agency
9 Croft Road
Bankend
Dumfries DG1 4RW
Tel.: 01387 770404 (helpline open Tuesday evenings only, 7 p.m. to 10 p.m.)
Text 07768 079 909
Website www.over-count.org.uk
A self-help group for people who have become addicted to over-the-counter medicines. Emails may be sent at any time but responses will only be given on Tuesdays.

Other groups, covering codeine overuse specifically, are at <www.codeinefree.com> and <www.codeinefree.me.uk>

Thoughtful Products
11 Willow Drive
Ripley
Surrey GU23 6LF
Tel.: 01483 224653
Website: www.thoughtfulproducts.co.uk
Provides aids such as the Loo Stool, which may help prevent constipation and alleviate prolapse.

Women's Health Concern Ltd
4–6 Eton Place
Marlow
Bucks SL7 2QA
Tel.: 01628 478 473
Website: www.womens-health-concern.org
This charity, established in 1972, offers information, including a confidential email advice line staffed by nurses and medical advisers. Alternatively, write to Confidential Advice Service at the above address.

Yes Pure Intimacy
3L Trading
PO Box 214
Alton
Hants GU34 3WY
Tel.: 0845 094 1141
Website: www.yesyesyes.org
Organic personal lubricants, made without chemicals such as parabens and hormones.

Yoga Biomedical Trust
Tel.: 020 8245 6420
Website: www.yogatherapy.org
This charitable trust, based in London, teaches yoga techniques to individuals for managing health problems and provides further training for yoga teachers.

USA

Estronaut
Website www.estronaut.com
A women's health site set up by a woman doctor.

George Mateljan Foundation for the World's Healthiest Foods
Website: www.whfoods.com
Detailed information about numerous foods, based on scientific evidence.

HERS Foundation
422 Bryn Mawr Avenue
Bala Cynwyd
Pennsylvania 19004
Tel.: (610) 667-7757
Website: www.hersfoundation.com
An independent non-profit international women's health education organization, it emphasizes hysterectomy's adverse effects and alternatives.

HysterSisters
Website: www.hystersisters.com
An online patient support group for women who have had or are about to have a hysterectomy. Also sells useful products such as the Swelly Belly Band, which can relieve post-operative discomfort and itching.

Inquisitive Geek with Fibroid Tumors
Website: http://blog. geekwithfibroids.com
A blogsite, run by a woman who keeps up with research into the subject, where women can share their experiences.

Whole Woman Center
418 Central Avenue SE
Albuquerque
New Mexico 87102
Tel.: 505-243-4010
Website: www.wholewoman.com
A site promoting alternative treatments, including self-help, for uterine prolapse and urinary incontinence.

Index